FIRST EDITION

Interventional Pain Procedure Templates

Procedure Notes Templates for Pain Physicians

to Simplify Data Entry

DR. PRIYA SADAWARTE, MD, DNB

MedMantra, LLC

New Mexico

First Edition of "Interventional Pain Procedure Templates"

by Dr. Priya Sadawarte, MD, DNB

Published by MedMantra, LLC

1330 San Pedro Drive NE STE 205A, Albuquerque, NM 87110

https://MedMantra.com

ISBN: 978-1-954612-04-4 (Paperback)

ISBN: 978-1-954612-05-1 (eBook)

Library of Congress Control Number: 2021932348 | Permalink: https://lccn.loc.gov/2021932348

Copyright © 2021 MedMantra, LLC

Register your copy:

First edition: February, 2021

Register your copy of this book by following the instructions mentioned at: https://MedMantra.com/ippt

Registration entitles you to a completely free eBook of the next edition.

Speaker invitations and business consultation requests:

Contact the author by email (drpriyasadawarte@gmail.com) for speaker invitations or business consultation requests.

DEDICATION

I would like to thank my parents; who gave me freedom to pursue whatever I wished. My in-laws; who always supported me whole-heartedly. I wish to thank my supportive husband, Sachin, and my two loving sons, Tanuj and Ojas, who provide unending inspiration. Most importantly, I want to thank my chronic pain patients, who inspire me to work harder by telling me how wonderful it feels to lead an active pain-free life.

Claim Your Surprise Gift

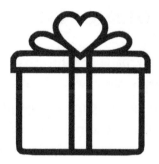

Thank you for checking out my book. To show my appreciation, I've prepared a special gift for all my readers that will help you write great procedure notes. The gift is in the form of electronic templates, procedure videos, training courses, and lots more...

Access it by visiting: **https://medmantra.com/ippt**

TABLE OF CONTENTS

SECTION 1
GENERAL CONSIDERATIONS

CHAPTER 1

BEFORE ENTERING PROCEDURE ROOM

- Assess patient's symptoms and examine him/her again before a planned procedure. Document your findings.

- Confirm pain location and laterality.

- Rule out allergies.

- Review current medications (especially anti-coagulants) and recent imaging.

- Explain the procedure in detail.

- While taking consent, always explain **B**enefits of doing the procedure, **R**isks involved in the procedure, **A**lternative treatment options available and what may happen if procedure is **n**ot performed. Always explain in patient's language. (Template of Informed consent form is provided in Annexure)

- Set appropriate expectations about pain relief: When will pain relief start, how long will it last, how much pain relief may be achieved. Pain relief spectrum varies from complete resolution of pain to no change in symptoms. (e.g. After epidural injection, patient will experience some immediate relief for a few hours due to local anesthetic drug, but patient may experience a brief recurrence of former pain until the anti-inflammatory medication takes effect. Pain will be relieved after a few days and may last for 6 months.)

- Enquire about results of prior injections. (if any)

- Get Complete blood count (CBC), Blood glucose level, bleeding time (BT), clotting time (CT), Prothrombin time (PT), International normalized ratio (INR), and S creatinine.

- Interventional pain procedures should be done in operating room or procedure room equipped with monitoring and resuscitation facility.

CHAPTER 2

BEFORE STARTING PROCEDURE

- Display recent imaging in procedure room view box.

- Confirm availability of resuscitation equipment and all the equipment needed for the procedure before starting procedure.

- Monitor Pulse, Non-invasive blood pressure, Oxygen saturation (SPO2), ECG throughout the procedure.

- Confirm that written informed consent is signed.

- Some of the procedures require patient to be NPO (6 hours for solids and 2 hours for clear fluids).

- Secure IV line.

- Some of the procedures require antibiotic cover.

- Most of the procedures can be done under Monitored Anesthesia Care (MAC). But, some of the procedures require sedation, some require Total intravenous anesthesia (TIVA).

- Always have an anesthesiologist standby.

- Radioprotection in the form of lead apron and thyroid shield is necessary. Using radiation counter is also preferable. For additional protection, radiation gloves and goggles may be used while doing a procedure.

- When positioning patient prone, position the target side away from you so that image intensifier is away from you when you are working. Position monitor at eye level on opposite side. Ergonomic placement is important.

- Be sure to rotate the on-screen image so that the patient's left is on screen left to reflect prone positioning.

- Aseptic precautions should be followed strictly. It includes wearing sterile gown and sterile gloves.

- Injection area should be cleaned thoroughly with betadine-spirit/ Chlorhexidine and draped with sterile fenestrated drape.

CHAPTER 3

DURING PROCEDURE

- It's important to learn to co-relate anatomy, surface anatomy and Fluoroanatomy

- After marking the entry point, advance the needle in tunnel vision

- Always check depth of insertion using intermittent fluoroscopy and confirm final position of needle tip in both AP and lateral view

- Always aspirate before injecting radiocontrast, local anesthetic, steroid and neurolytic agent.

- Always inject radiocontrast in real-time fluoroscopy, otherwise vascular spread may be missed.

- Attach a 10 cm connection to the needle before injecting radiocontrast, to avoid radio-exposure to hands while injecting in real-time fluoroscopy

- Always save an image of radiocontrast spread. If possible, print and attach a copy to procedure notes.

- Inject local anesthetic before radiofrequency lesioning and neurolytic injection to reduce pain.

- After injecting neurolytic, flush the syringe with local anesthetic solution while withdrawing. This reduces post-procedure pain at the injection site.

- During epidural, when you are close to the neural foramen, inform the patient that they may experience radicular symptoms.

- Once in the epidural space, inject the steroid slowly. Warn the patient they may experience radicular symptoms as the steroid solution fills the foramen and bathes the nerve roots. If patient experiences radicular symptoms, stop injecting for some time and then inject at a lower rate of injection. It is important to deposit the medication into the epidural space, but it's immaterial how quickly it goes in.

- After the injection is complete, inform the patient that you are removing the needle and do so slowly.

- After removing the needle, cleanse the skin thoroughly with isopropyl alcohol-soaked gauze (residual betadine may cause itching). Confirm that needle/catheter is removed intact.

- Remove the drapes and place a band-aid at the puncture site.

- Ask the patient sit up on the procedure table for few minutes (unless patient has received TIVA). Ensure that they are not light-headed or dizzy.

- Warn patients about possibility of limb weakness, wherever it's a possibility. Explain that it will last only 1-2 hours. When the patient is ready, assist them step off the table and start weightbearing. Shift the patient to recovery room in a wheel chair/stretcher.

CHAPTER 4

AFTER PROCEDURE

- Ask patient to rest, lying down, in a recovery room for 30 minutes to few hours.

- Blood pressure, pulse, respiration, Oxygen saturation should be monitored in recovery room. Document the vital signs. Additional neurological/ temperature monitoring should be done wherever necessary

- Patient should be accompanied by a responsible adult.

- Explain activity limitations post procedure: Patient must not drive himself/herself after few procedures e.g. after lumbar epidural injection. He/she should take it easy the remainder of the day, can return to routine activity the following day. (in most of the procedures)

- Fix a follow-up appointment

CHAPTER 5

DISCHARGE INSTRUCTIONS

- Apply ice to the injection area to decrease discomfort.

- Do not drive or operate machinery for at least 24 hours after certain procedures like lumbar epidural injection.

- You may eat your normal diet. (For most of the procedures)

- Do not participate in strenuous activity that day.

- You may remove any bandages the morning following the procedure.

- You may take a shower. Do not sit in a hot tub for 24 hours.

- Post-procedure, ask the patient to maintain a pain diary

- If you are taking a blood thinner like aspirin, Clopidogrel, Ticlopidine, warfarin, heparin, LMWH among others, please restart only after confirming with your doctor.

- If you develop a fever, chills, breathing difficulty, increasing pain, or if you have new symptoms, please call your physician's office directly (Provide an emergency contact number.)

Communicating with patient is the key!

Section 2

Spine:

Cervical/Thoracic/
Lumbar/Sacral

CHAPTER 1

CERVICAL INTERLAMINAR EPIDURAL INJECTION

Name: _____ age/sex _____ date/time _____

PROCEDURE: Cervical interlaminar epidural injection under fluoroscopy guidance, _____ level, left/right side

DIAGNOSIS: _____

PHYSICIAN: _____

MEDICATIONS INJECTED: 2 ml of Dexamethasone (8 mg) and 4 ml 0.125% Bupivacaine

ANAESTHESIA: Local/sedation/TIVA/General Anesthesia

SEDATION MEDICATIONS: None

COMPLICATIONS: None

TECHNIQUE: After confirming written informed consent and NPO status, multipara monitor was attached to the patient. Intravenous access was secured. Time-out was taken to identify the correct patient, procedure and side prior to starting the procedure.

Patient was placed in Prone position, with a pillow under upper chest for neck flexion. Parts were prepped and draped in the usual sterile fashion using betadine-spirit and sterile fenestrated drape. C6-C7/ C7-T1 level was determined under fluoroscopy in AP view. End plate was squared. Entry point was marked at the lamina, midway between the pedicle and spinous process. Local anesthetic 3 ml of 1% Lignocaine was given by raising a skin wheal and in subcutaneous tissue along path of Touhy needle using a 26-gauge 1.25-inch needle.

The 18-gauge, 3.5-inch Tuohy needle was introduced at the entry point and advanced perpendicular to skin, in tunnel view, to contact lamina. Then it was walked off the lamina. Stylet was removed, and LOR syringe was attached. (LOR to air/saline) Needle was advanced slowly. After feeling loss of resistance for ligamentum flavum, epidural space was again confirmed with hanging drop method. C-arm was turned contra lateral oblique to confirm that needle tip was posterior to spino-laminar line.

1 ml Omnipaque 240 was injected in real time fluoroscopy to confirm epidural position of needle tip. Honeycomb appearance and Christmas tree appearance was seen on AP view. Contrast spread was seen at spino-laminar line in contralateral oblique view. There was no vascular runoff. Treatment medication was then injected slowly in 1 ml aliquots. Needle was removed intact. A sterile dressing was applied.

The procedure was completed without complications and was tolerated well. After the procedure, the patient was monitored for 60 minutes in the recovery room. The patient (or responsible adult) was given post-procedure and discharge instructions to follow at home. The patient was discharged in stable condition after making a follow-up appointment.

Pre-procedure pain score: _____

Post-procedure pain score: _____

CHAPTER 2

CERVICAL INTERLAMINAR EPIDURAL INJECTION WITH EPIDURAL CATHERTERISATION

Name: _____ age/sex _____ date/time _____

PROCEDURE: Cervical interlaminar epidural injection with epidural catheterization under fluoroscopy guidance, _____ level, left/right side

DIAGNOSIS: _____

PHYSICIAN: _____

MEDICATIONS INJECTED: 2 ml of Dexamethasone (8 mg) and 4 ml 0.125% Bupivacaine

ANAESTHESIA: Local/sedation/TIVA/General Anesthesia

SEDATION MEDICATIONS: None

COMPLICATIONS: None

TECHNIQUE: After confirming written informed consent and NPO status, multipara monitor was attached to the patient. Intravenous access was secured. Time-out was taken to identify the correct patient, procedure and side prior to starting the procedure.

Patient was placed in prone position, with a pillow under upper chest for neck flexion. Parts were prepped and draped in the usual sterile fashion using betadine, spirit and sterile fenestrated drape. C6-C7/C7-T1 level was determined under fluoroscopy in AP view. End plate was squared. Entry point was marked at the lamina, midway between the pedicle and spinous process. Local anesthetic 5 ml of 1% Lignocaine was given by raising a skin wheal and in subcutaneous tissue along path of Touhy needle using a 26-gauge 1.25-inch needle.

An 18-gauge, 3.5-inch Tuohy needle was introduced at the entry point and advanced perpendicular to skin, in tunnel view, to contact lamina. Then it was walked off the lamina. Stylet was removed, and LOR syringe was attached. (LOR to air/saline) Needle was advanced slowly. After feeling loss of resistance for ligamentum flavum, epidural space was again confirmed with hanging drop method. C-arm was turned contra lateral oblique to confirm that needle tip was posterior to spino-laminar line. Epidural catheter was then inserted up to .... mark to reach desired level.

1 ml Omnipaque 240 was injected in real time fluoroscopy through the catheter to confirm epidural position of catheter tip. Honeycomb appearance was seen on AP view. Contrast spread was seen at spino-laminar line in contralateral oblique view. There was no vascular runoff. Treatment medication was then injected slowly in 1 ml aliquots. Needle and catheter were removed intact. A sterile dressing was applied.

The procedure was completed without complications and was tolerated well. After the procedure, the patient was monitored for 60 minutes in the recovery room. The patient (or responsible adult) was given post-procedure and discharge instructions to follow at home. The patient was discharged in stable condition after making a follow-up appointment.

Pre-procedure pain score: _____

Post-procedure pain score: _____

CHAPTER 3

DIAGNOSTIC CERVICAL MEDIAL BRANCH BLOCK (MBB) IN PRONE POSITION

Name: _____ age/sex _____ date/time _____

PROCEDURE: Diagnostic Cervical Medial Branch block in prone position under Fluoroscopic guidance, _____ level, left/right side

DIAGNOSIS: _____

PHYSICIAN: _____

MEDICATIONS INJECTED: 0.5 ml of 2% Lignocaine/ 0.25% Bupivacaine

ANAESTHESIA: Local/sedation/TIVA/General Anesthesia

SEDATION MEDICATIONS: None

COMPLICATIONS: None

TECHNIQUE: After confirming written informed consent and NPO status, multipara monitor was attached to the patient. Intravenous access was secured. Time-out was taken to identify the correct patient, procedure and side prior to starting the procedure. Patient was positioned prone with cervical spine flexed by keeping pillow under chest, arms by the side. Parts were prepped and draped in the usual sterile fashion using betadine-spirit and sterile fenestrated drape. Desired levels were determined on fluoroscopy in AP view. Image intensifier was rotated caudal to align it with axis of orientation of facet joints, facet joints are seen as transverse lines. Entry point was marked at the lateral aspect of midportion of lamina. (For C7 MBB, entry point was marked at the junction of superior articular process and transverse process of C7). Local anesthetic 5 ml of 1% Lignocaine was given at each site by raising a skin wheal and along path of the needle using a 26-gauge 1.25-inch needle.

The 25-gauge 1.5-inch hypodermic needle was inserted at the entry point and advanced in tunnel view utilizing intermittent fluoroscopy till it made bony contact. Needle position was confirmed to be at lateral aspect of midportion lamina on AP view and center of articular process on lateral view. Treatment medication was then injected slowly. Similar procedure was repeated at each desired level. Needles were removed intact. A sterile dressing was applied.

The procedure was completed without complications and was tolerated well. After the procedure, the patient was monitored for 30 minutes in the recovery room. The patient (or responsible adult) was given post-procedure and discharge instructions to follow at home. The patient was discharged in stable condition after making a follow-up appointment.

Note: Patient was instructed to maintain a pain diary after the block. The patient was also instructed to do the activities that would normally worsen the pain. He/she was asked to note percentage of pain relief obtained at rest and after activity and also duration of pain relief.

Pre-procedure pain score: _____

Post-procedure pain score: _____

Note: Each cervical facet is innervated by two medial branches. e.g., C4-C5 facet joint is innervated by C4 and C5 medial branches. Only exception is C2-C3 facet joint, innervated by medial branch from C3 only (third occipital nerve).

CHAPTER 4

DIAGNOSTIC CERVICAL MEDIAL BRANCH BLOCK(MBB) IN LATERAL POSITION

Name: _____ age/sex _____date/time _____

PROCEDURE: Diagnostic Cervical Medial Branch block in lateral position under Fluoroscopic guidance, _____ level, left/right side

DIAGNOSIS: _____

PHYSICIAN: _____

MEDICATIONS INJECTED: 0.5 ml of 2% Lignocaine/ 0.25% Bupivacaine

ANAESTHESIA: Local/sedation/TIVA/General Anesthesia

SEDATION MEDICATIONS: None

COMPLICATIONS: None

TECHNIQUE: After confirming written informed consent and NPO status, multipara monitor was attached to the patient. Intravenous access was secured. Time-out was taken to identify the correct patient, procedure and side prior to starting the procedure. Patient was positioned lateral with a pillow under head and neck slightly flexed. Patient was asked to hold flexed knees with hands. Parts were prepped and draped in the usual sterile fashion using betadine-spirit and sterile fenestrated drape. Desired levels were determined on fluoroscopy in lateral image of cervical spine. Image intensifier was rotated right-left oblique to superimpose the articular processes at the desired level to eliminate vertical parallax. Then image intensifier was rotated cephalic-caudal to superimpose facet joint lines to eliminate horizontal parallax. Crisp rhomboid image of the articular pillars of the desired level was obtained. Entry point was marked at centroid of the articular pillar. Local anesthetic 5 ml of 1% Lignocaine was given at each site by raising a skin wheal and along path of the needle using a 26-gauge 1.25-inch needle.

The 25-gauge 1.5-inch hypodermic needle was inserted at the entry point and advanced in tunnel view utilizing intermittent fluoroscopy till it made bony contact. Needle position was confirmed to be at centroid of articular process on lateral image of cervical spine and at the lateral aspect of midportion lamina on AP image of cervical spine. Needle was withdrawn by 1 mm and treatment medication was then injected slowly after negative aspiration. Similar procedure was repeated at each desired level. Needles were removed intact. A sterile dressing was applied.

The procedure was completed without complications and was tolerated well. After the procedure, the patient was monitored for 30 minutes in the recovery room. The patient (or responsible adult) was given post-procedure and discharge instructions to follow at home. The patient was discharged in stable condition after making a follow-up appointment.

Note: Patient was instructed to maintain a pain diary after the block. The patient was also instructed to do the activities that would normally worsen the pain. He/she was asked to note percentage of pain relief obtained at rest and after activity and also duration of pain relief.

Pre-procedure pain score: _____

Post-procedure pain score: _____

CHAPTER 5

CERVICAL MEDIAL BRANCH
RADIOFREQUENCY ABLATION

Name: _____ age/sex _____date/time _____

PROCEDURE: Cervical Medial branch radiofrequency ablation under Fluoroscopic guidance, _____ level, left/right side

DIAGNOSIS: _____

PHYSICIAN: _____

MEDICATIONS INJECTED: Before ablation, 0.5 ml of 1% Lignocaine at each level. After ablation, 1 ml of 1% Lignocaine at each site

ANAESTHESIA: Local/sedation/TIVA/General Anesthesia

SEDATION MEDICATIONS: None

COMPLICATIONS: None

TECHNIQUE: After confirming written informed consent and NPO status, multipara monitor was attached to the patient. Intravenous access was secured. Time-out was taken to identify the correct patient, procedure and side prior to starting the procedure.

Patient was positioned prone with cervical spine flexed by keeping pillow under chest. Parts were prepped and draped in the usual sterile fashion using betadine-spirit and sterile fenestrated drape. Desired levels were determined under fluoroscopy in AP view. C-arm was rotated caudal to align it with axis of orientation of facet joints. Entry point was marked at middle of articular pillar at the desired level. (For C7 level, entry point was marked at the junction of superior articular process and transverse process of C7) Local anesthetic 3 ml of 1% Lignocaine was given at each site by raising a skin wheal and along path of radiofrequency needle using a 26-gauge 1.25-inch needle.

A 20-gauge, curved, 100 mm radiofrequency needle with 5 mm active tip was inserted at the entry point and advanced to the anatomic location of the medial branch at the lateral masses utilizing intermittent fluoroscopy. Needle is advanced till it reaches the lateral border between superior and inferior articulating surfaces. Needle tip was walked off the lateral edge of the vertebral body about 2-3 mm so that active tip was positioned parallel to the medial branch nerve. Needle tip was confirmed to be posterior to the posterior margin of neural foramen in lateral view. Sensory stimulation at 50 Hz was applied at each level, paresthesia was noted at 0.3-0.5 V. Motor stimulation at 2Hz up to 2 volts was applied at each level which showed no extremity movement. 0.5 ml of 1% Lignocaine was then injected slowly at each level. After waiting 30-60 seconds, ablation was performed utilizing a radiofrequency generator at 60^0 C for 60 seconds. The needles were then withdrawn by 5mm and rotated. Then a second ablation was done at 60^0 C for another 60 seconds. After the ablation, 1 ml of 1% Lignocaine was injected at each site as the needles were removed to numb the track. Needles were removed intact. A sterile dressing was applied.

The procedure was completed without complications and was tolerated well. After the procedure, the patient was monitored for 2 hours in the recovery room. The patient (or responsible adult) was given post-procedure and discharge instructions to follow at home. The patient was discharged in stable condition after making a follow-up appointment.

Pre-procedure pain score: _____

Post-procedure pain score: _____

CHAPTER 6

DIAGNOSTIC T2-T3 SYMPATHETIC BLOCK

Name: _____ age/sex _____ date/time _____

PROCEDURE: Diagnostic T2-T3 sympathetic block under Fluoroscopic guidance, left/right side

DIAGNOSIS: _____

PHYSICIAN: _____

MEDICATIONS INJECTED: 5 ml of 0.25% Bupivacaine with 20 mg Methylprednisolone/ Triamcinolone at each level.

SEDATION MEDICATIONS: None

ANAESTHESIA: Local/sedation/TIVA/General Anesthesia

COMPLICATIONS: None

TECHNIQUE: After confirming written informed consent and NPO status, multipara monitor was attached to the patient. Surface thermometry probe was attached on both the upper extremities. Intravenous access was secured. Time-out was taken to identify the correct patient, procedure and side prior to starting the procedure.

With the patient lying in the prone position, parts were prepped and draped in the usual sterile fashion using betadine-spirit and sterile fenestrated drape. Using AP view on fluoroscopy, T2 vertebra was identified. Superior endplate of T2 vertebra was squared by moving image intensifier cephalad and then it was rotated ipsilateral oblique. Entry point was marked at the lateral edge of T2 vertebral body on desired side, just cephalad to third rib. Entry point was .... cm from T2 spinous process on surface anatomy. Local anesthetic was given in skin and subcutaneous tissue using 25-gauge 1.25-inch needle.

23-gauge 10 cm spinal needle with curved tip was inserted at the entry point and advanced in a tunnel view towards lateral border of T2 vertebral body, above third rib. Needle was advanced under intermittent AP and lateral fluoroscopy. After needle tip hit vertebral body, needle was rotated by 90^0 to slip off the vertebral body. Final position of needle was confirmed to be at the posterior third of midline in cephalo-caudad relation of vertebral body on lateral view. 1 ml of radiocontrast was injected after aspiration. Linear spread along the anterior border of thoracic vertebral column was seen on lateral view and vacuolated appearance was seen in AP view with no vascular uptake. Needle aspiration was performed and medication was then injected slowly. Similar procedure was repeated at T3 level. Needles were removed intact. A sterile dressing was applied.

The procedure was completed without complications and was tolerated well. After the procedure, the patient was monitored for 2 hours in the recovery room. Monitoring was done for hemodynamic stability, Skin temperature, Sensory and motor function of upper extremity, Vasodilation, change of color, decreased sweating, and pain reduction. The patient (or responsible adult) was given post-procedure and discharge instructions to follow at home. The patient was discharged in stable condition after making a follow-up appointment

Right upper extremity: Pre-injection skin temp = _____ Post-injection skin temp= _____

Left upper extremity: Pre-injection skin temp= _____ Post-injection skin temp= _____

Pre-procedure pain score: _____

Post-procedure pain score: _____

Note: Patient was instructed to maintain a pain diary after the block. The patient was also instructed to do the activities that would normally worsen the pain. He/she was asked to note percentage of pain relief obtained at rest and after activity and also duration of pain relief.

CHAPTER 7

T2-T3 SYMPATHETIC RADIOFREQUENCY ABLATION

Name: _____ age/sex _____ date/time _____

PROCEDURE: T2-T3 sympathetic radiofrequency ablation under Fluoroscopic guidance, left/right side

DIAGNOSIS: _____

PHYSICIAN: _____

MEDICATIONS INJECTED: 3 ml of 0.25% Bupivacaine with 20 mg Triamcinolone at each level

SEDATION MEDICATIONS: None

ANAESTHESIA: Local/sedation/TIVA/General Anesthesia

COMPLICATIONS: None

TECHNIQUE: After confirming written informed consent and NPO status, multipara monitor was attached to the patient. Surface thermometry probe was attached on both the upper extremities. Intravenous access was secured. Time-out was taken to identify the correct patient, procedure and side prior to starting the procedure.

With the patient lying in the prone position, parts were prepped and draped in the usual sterile fashion using betadine-spirit and sterile fenestrated drape. Using AP view on fluoroscopy, T2 vertebra was identified. Superior endplate of T2 vertebra was squared by moving image intensifier cephalad and ipsilateral oblique. Entry point was marked at the lateral edge of T2 vertebral body, just cephalad to third rib. Entry point was ....cm from T2 spinous process on surface anatomy. Local anesthetic was given in skin and subcutaneous tissue using 25-gauge 1.25-inch needle.

22-gauge 100mm curved tip Radiofrequency needle with 10 mm active tip was inserted at the entry point and advanced in a tunnel view towards lateral border of T2 vertebral body, above third rib. Needle was advanced under intermittent AP and lateral fluoroscopy. After needle tip hit vertebral body, needle was rotated by 90^0 to slip off the vertebral body. Final position of needle was confirmed to be at the posterior third of midline in cephalo-caudad relation of vertebral body on lateral view. 1 ml of radiocontrast was injected after aspiration. Linear spread along the anterior border of thoracic vertebral column was seen on lateral view and vacuolated appearance was seen in AP view with no vascular uptake. On sensory stimulation with 50 Hz up to 0.6 V, there was no dermatome related sensation. On motor stimulation at 2Hz up to 1.2 V, there was no intercostal muscle contraction. 1 ml of 1% Lignocaine was then injected slowly. After waiting 30-60 seconds, ablation was performed utilizing a radiofrequency generator at 80^0 C for 60 seconds. The needles were then withdrawn by 5mm and rotated. Then a second ablation was done at 80^0 C for 60 seconds. After the ablation, needle aspiration was performed and medication was injected slowly. Similar procedure was repeated at T3 level. Needles were removed intact. A sterile dressing was applied.

The procedure was completed without complications and was tolerated well. After the procedure, the patient was monitored for 2 hours in the recovery room. Monitoring was done for hemodynamic stability, Skin temperature, Sensory/ motor function of upper extremity, Vasodilation, change of color, decreased sweating, and pain reduction. The patient (or responsible adult) was given post-procedure and discharge instructions to follow at home. The patient was discharged in stable condition after making a follow-up appointment

Right upper extremity: Pre-injection skin temp = _____ Post-injection skin temp=_____

Left upper extremity: Pre-injection skin temp= _____ Post-injection skin temp= _____

Pre-procedure pain score: _____

Post-procedure pain score: _____

CHAPTER 8

LUMBAR EPIDURAL INJECTION: TRANSFORAMINAL

Name: _____ age/sex _____ date/time _____

PROCEDURE: Fluoroscopy guided transforaminal epidural injection, _____ level, left/right side

DIAGNOSIS: _____

PHYSICIAN: _____

MEDICATIONS INJECTED: 2 ml of 0.125% Bupivacaine with 20 mg Methylprednisolone/Triamcinolone

ANAESTHESIA: Local/sedation/TIVA/General Anesthesia

SEDATION MEDICATIONS: None

COMPLICATIONS: None

TECHNIQUE: After confirming written informed consent and NPO status, multipara monitor was attached to the patient. Intravenous access was secured. Time-out was taken to identify the correct patient, procedure and side prior to starting the procedure.

With the patient lying in the prone position and pillow under abdomen, parts were prepped and draped in the usual sterile fashion using betadine-spirit and sterile fenestrated drape. Desired vertebral levels were identified on AP view. Squaring of the endplates was done by rotating image intensifier caudally. Then it was rotated oblique ipsilaterally till medial border of pedicle was in line with lateral border of lamina. Scotty dog appearance was seen. Local anesthetic 5 ml of 1% Lignocaine was given at 6 o'clock position of the pedicle at each desired site by raising a skin wheal and along path of Quincke needle using a 26-gauge 1.25-inch needle.

3.5-inch 23-gauge Quincke needle with curved tip was used. In an ipsilateral oblique view needle was inserted with curve medially at 6 o'clock position of the pedicle. The needle was advanced in tunnel view via intermittent fluoroscopic imaging. It was advanced till it made bony contact with the pedicle. Then curve was turned laterally and needle was advanced. A give-way was felt. Needle tip was seen just below the midpoint of pedicle, not crossing facet joint line on AP view and in the postero-superior quadrant of neural foramen in lateral view. After attaching 10 cm connection to the needle, 2 ml of Omnipaque 240 was injected in real-time fluoroscopy. It was seen along medial and inferior side of pedicle in AP view and along the spino-laminar line in lateral view, thus confirming epidural spread. There was no vascular runoff. After a negative aspiration, the medication was injected slowly. Needle was removed intact. A sterile dressing was applied.

The procedure was completed without complications and was tolerated well. After the procedure, the patient was monitored for 30 minutes in the recovery room. The patient (or responsible adult) was given post-procedure and discharge instructions to follow at home. The patient was discharged in stable condition after making a follow-up appointment.

Pre-procedure pain score: _____

Post-procedure pain score: _____

CHAPTER 9

LUMBAR EPIDURAL INJECTION: INTERLAMINAR

Name: _____ age/sex _____ date/time _____

PROCEDURE: Lumbar interlaminar epidural injection under fluoroscopy guidance, _____ level, left/right side

DIAGNOSIS: _____

PHYSICIAN: _____

MEDICATIONS INJECTED: 1 ml of Methylprednisolone/Triamcinolone (40 mg) and 5 ml 0.125% Bupivacaine

ANAESTHESIA: Local/sedation/TIVA/General Anesthesia

SEDATION MEDICATIONS: None

COMPLICATIONS: None

TECHNIQUE: After confirming written informed consent and NPO status, multipara monitor was attached to the patient. Intravenous access was secured. Time-out was taken to identify the correct patient, procedure and side prior to starting the procedure.

Patient was placed in Prone position, with a pillow under abdomen. Parts were prepped and draped in the usual sterile fashion using betadine-spirit and sterile fenestrated drape. Desired level was determined under fluoroscopy in AP view. End plates were squared by rotating the image intensifier caudally. Entry point was marked at the superior border of lower lamina, midway between the pedicle and spinous process. Local anesthetic 3 ml of 1% Lignocaine was given by raising a skin wheal and in subcutaneous tissue along path of Touhy needle using a 26-gauge 1.25-inch needle.

The 18-gauge, 3.5-inch Tuohy needle was introduced at the entry point and advanced perpendicular to skin, in tunnel view, to contact superior border of lower lamina. Then it was walked off the lamina. Stylet was removed, and LOR syringe was attached. Needle was advanced slowly using LOR to air/saline. After feeling loss of resistance for ligamentum flavum, epidural space was again confirmed with hanging drop method. C-arm was turned lateral to confirm that needle tip was posterior to spino-laminar line.

2 ml Omnipaque 240 was injected to confirm epidural position of needle tip. Honeycomb appearance was seen on AP view. Contrast spread was seen at spino-laminar line in lateral view. There was no vascular runoff. Treatment medication was then injected slowly. Needle was removed intact. A sterile dressing was applied.

The procedure was completed without complications and was tolerated well. After the procedure, the patient was monitored for 30 minutes in the recovery room. The patient (or responsible adult) was given post-procedure and discharge instructions to follow at home. The patient was discharged in stable condition after making a follow-up appointment.

Pre-procedure pain score: _____

Post-procedure pain score: _____

CHAPTER 10

CAUDAL EPIDURAL INJECTION

Name: _____ age/sex _____date/time _____

PROCEDURE: Caudal epidural injection under Fluoroscopic guidance

DIAGNOSIS: _____

PHYSICIAN: _____

MEDICATIONS INJECTED: 12 ml of 0.25% Bupivacaine/ 1% Lignocaine with 20 mg Triamcinolone/Methylprednisolone

ANAESTHESIA: Local/sedation/TIVA/General Anesthesia

SEDATION MEDICATIONS: None

COMPLICATIONS: None

TECHNIQUE: After confirming written informed consent and NPO status, multipara monitor was attached to the patient. Intravenous access was secured. Time-out was taken to identify the correct patient, procedure and side prior to starting the procedure.

With the patient lying in the prone position with pillow under lower abdomen, parts were prepped and draped in the usual sterile fashion using betadine-spirit and sterile fenestrated drape. Sacral hiatus was palpated, and also identified on AP view and lateral view in fluoroscopy. Local anesthetic 5 ml of 1% Lignocaine was given by raising a skin wheal and in subcutaneous tissue using a 26-gauge 1.25-inch needle.

Under fluoroscopic guidance, a 23-gauge 3.5-inch Quincke needle was inserted in lateral view and advanced cephalad towards sacral hiatus at 45⁰ angles. Sacrococcygeal ligament was penetrated and loss of resistance was felt. On lateral view, when needle was seen touching posterior sacral plate, needle bevel was turned anterior and advanced to enter sacral canal. Correct needle placement was confirmed by both AP and lateral fluoroscopy. After negative aspiration, administration of 0.5 ml of the contrast revealed correct needle placement within the sacral canal. There was neither intravascular nor intradural uptake. An additional 4 ml of contrast was administered, revealing additional epidural flow up to L5-S1. After negative aspiration, treatment medication was injected slowly. The needle was removed intact. A sterile dressing was applied.

The procedure was completed without complications and was tolerated well. After the procedure, the patient was monitored for 30 minutes in the recovery room. The patient (or responsible adult) was given post-procedure and discharge instructions to follow at home. The patient was discharged in stable condition after making a follow-up appointment.

Pre-procedure pain score: _____

Post-procedure pain score: _____

CHAPTER 11

CAUDAL EPIDURAL INJECTION
WITH CATHETERIZATION

Name: _____ age/sex _____ date/time _____

PROCEDURE: Caudal epidural injection with catheterization under Fluoroscopic guidance, catheter up to _____ level

DIAGNOSIS: _____

PHYSICIAN: _____

MEDICATIONS INJECTED: 4 ml of 0.25% Bupivacaine/ 1% Lignocaine with 20 mg Triamcinolone/Methylprednisolone

ANAESTHESIA: Local/sedation/TIVA/General Anesthesia

SEDATION MEDICATIONS: None

COMPLICATIONS: None

TECHNIQUE: After confirming written informed consent and NPO status, multipara monitor was attached to the patient. Intravenous access was secured. Time-out was taken to identify the correct patient, procedure and side prior to starting the procedure.

With the patient lying in the prone position with pillow under lower abdomen, parts were prepped and draped in the usual sterile fashion using betadine-spirit and sterile fenestrated drape. Sacral hiatus was palpated, and also identified on AP view and lateral view in fluoroscopy. Local anesthetic 5 ml of 1% Lignocaine was given at entry point by raising a skin wheal and in subcutaneous tissue using a 26-gauge 1.25-inch needle.

Under fluoroscopic guidance, an 18-gauge Touhy needle was inserted in lateral view and advanced cephalad towards sacral hiatus at 45⁰ angles. Sacrococcygeal ligament was penetrated and loss of resistance was felt. On lateral view, when needle was seen touching posterior sacral plate, needle bevel was turned anterior and advanced to enter sacral canal. Correct needle placement was confirmed by both AP and lateral fluoroscopy. After negative aspiration, administration of 0.5 ml of the contrast revealed correct needle placement within the sacral canal. There was neither intravascular nor intradural uptake. Catheter was inserted up to the required level. An additional 1 ml of contrast was administered, revealing epidural flow. After negative aspiration, treatment medication was injected slowly. The needle and catheter were removed intact. A sterile dressing was applied.

The procedure was completed without complications and was tolerated well. After the procedure, the patient was monitored for 30 minutes in the recovery room. The patient (or responsible adult) was given post-procedure and discharge instructions to follow at home. The patient was discharged in stable condition after making a follow-up appointment.

Pre-procedure pain score: _____

Post-procedure pain score: _____

CHAPTER 12

LUMBAR FACET JOINT INJECTION

Name: _____ age/sex _____ date/time _____

PROCEDURE: Fluoroscopy guided facet joint injection, _____ level, left/right side

DIAGNOSIS: _____

PHYSICIAN: _____

MEDICATIONS INJECTED: 0.5 ml of 0.125% Bupivacaine with 0.5 ml (20mg) Methylprednisolone/Triamcinolone

ANAESTHESIA: Local/sedation/TIVA/General Anesthesia

SEDATION MEDICATIONS: None

COMPLICATIONS: None

TECHNIQUE: After confirming written informed consent and NPO status, multipara monitor was attached to the patient. Intravenous access was secured. Time-out was taken to identify the correct patient, procedure and side prior to starting the procedure.

With the patient lying in the prone position with pillow under abdomen, the parts were prepped and draped in the usual sterile fashion using betadine-spirit and sterile fenestrated drape. Desired levels were determined under fluoroscopy AP view. Image intensifier was rotated ipsilateral oblique till Scotty Dog appearance and open S-shaped facet joint space was seen. Entry point was marked just lateral to the inferior edge of Inferior Articular Process. Local anesthetic 5 ml of 1% Lignocaine was injected by raising a skin wheal and along path of Quincke needle using a 26-gauge 1.25-inch needle.

The 23-gauge 3.5-inch Quincke needle was inserted at the entry point and advanced in tunnel view. A pop was felt on entering the joint. After a negative aspiration to make sure that there was no intravascular placement, 0.5 ml Omnipaque 240 was injected in real-time fluoroscopy. Dumbbell shaped radiocontrast spread in oblique view and discoid shape in AP view confirmed intraarticular position. There was no vascular runoff. Treatment medication was then injected slowly. Needle was removed intact. A sterile dressing was applied.

The procedure was completed without complications and was tolerated well. After the procedure, the patient was monitored for 30 minutes in the recovery room. The patient (or responsible adult) was given post-procedure and discharge instructions to follow at home. The patient was discharged in stable condition after making a follow-up appointment.

Pre-procedure pain score: _____

Post-procedure pain score: _____

CHAPTER 13

DIAGNOSTIC LUMBAR MEDIAL BRANCH BLOCK (MBB)

Name: _____ age/sex _____ date/time _____

PROCEDURE: Diagnostic Lumbar Medial Branch block under Fluoroscopic guidance, _____ .level, left/right side

DIAGNOSIS: _____

PHYSICIAN: _____

MEDICATIONS INJECTED: 0.5 ml of 0.25% Bupivacaine/ 1% Lignocaine with 20 mg Triamcinolone/ Methylprednisolone

ANAESTHESIA: Local/sedation/TIVA/General Anesthesia

SEDATION MEDICATIONS: None

COMPLICATIONS: None

TECHNIQUE: After confirming written informed consent and NPO status, multipara monitor was attached to the patient. Intravenous access was secured. Time-out was taken to identify the correct patient, procedure and side prior to starting the procedure.

With the patient lying in the prone position with pillow under lower abdomen, parts were prepped and draped in the usual sterile fashion using betadine-spirit and sterile fenestrated drape. Desired level was identified in AP view. Then image intensifier was rotated ipsilateral oblique till Scotty Dog appearance was seen. A point at the junction of upper border of transverse process and Superior articular process was marked. (for L5, entry point at the junction of ala of sacrum and superior articular process of sacrum was marked) Local anesthetic 5 ml of 1% Lignocaine was given at each site by raising a skin wheal and along path of Quincke needle using a 26-gauge 1.25-inch needle.

The 23-gauge 3.5-inch Quincke needle was advanced to the anatomic location of each medial branch at the junction of the superior articular process and transverse process utilizing intermittent fluoroscopy. Needle was advanced in tunnel view till it made bony contact with the most medial end of superior edge of transverse process. Needle bevel was facing medially and inferiorly for L1-L4/ medially at L5. Needle tip position was checked in oblique and lateral view. 0.5 ml radiocontrast was injected. Medication was then injected slowly. The needle was removed intact. A sterile dressing was applied. Procedure was repeated at _____ levels. The procedure was completed without complications and was tolerated well. After the procedure, the patient was monitored for 30 minutes in the recovery room. The patient (or responsible adult) was given post-procedure and discharge instructions to follow at home. The patient was discharged in stable condition after making a follow-up appointment.

Note: The patient was instructed to maintain a pain diary every hour for 6 hours after the block. The patient was also instructed to do the activities that would normally worsen the pain. He/she was asked to note percentage of pain relief obtained at rest and after activity and also duration of pain relief.

Pre-procedure pain score: _____

Post-procedure pain score: _____

Note: for **L4-L5 facet joint** medial branches at L4 (at the level of transverse process of **L5 vertebral**) and L3 (at the level of transverse process of **L4 vertebra**) are blocked.

CHAPTER 14

LUMBAR MEDIAL BRANCH RADIOFREQUENCY ABLATION

Name: _____ age/sex _____date/time _____

PROCEDURE: Lumbar Medial branch radiofrequency ablation under Fluoroscopic guidance, _____.level, left/right side

DIAGNOSIS: _____

PHYSICIAN: _____

MEDICATIONS INJECTED: Before the ablation, 0.5 ml of 1% Lignocaine at each level. After the ablation, 1 ml (40mg) of Methylprednisolone/Triamcinolone divided between the radiofrequency sites. Also 2 ml of 0.125% Bupivacaine at each site

SEDATION MEDICATIONS: None

ANAESTHESIA: Local/sedation/TIVA/General Anesthesia

COMPLICATIONS: None

TECHNIQUE: After confirming written informed consent and NPO status, multipara monitor was attached to the patient. Intravenous access was secured. Time-out was taken to identify the correct patient, procedure and side prior to starting the procedure.

With the patient lying in the prone position with pillow under lower abdomen, parts were prepped and draped in the usual sterile fashion using betadine-spirit and sterile fenestrated drape. Desired level was identified in AP view. Then image intensifier was rotated ipsilateral oblique till Scotty Dog appearance was seen. A point at the junction of upper border of transverse process and Superior articular process was marked. (for L5, entry point at the junction of ala of sacrum and superior articular process of sacrum was marked). Local anesthetic 5 ml of 1% Lignocaine was given at each site by raising a skin wheal and along path of radiofrequency needle using a 26-gauge 1.25-inch needle.

A 20G 100mm radiofrequency needle with 10 mm active tip was introduced to the anatomic location of the medial branch at the junction of the superior articular process and transverse process utilizing intermittent fluoroscopy. Needle was advanced end-on till it made bony contact with the most medial end of superior edge of transverse process. Then needle is slid along the transverse process to lay it flat along target site. Needle bevel was facing medially and inferiorly for L1-L4/ medially at L5. Needle tip position was checked in oblique and lateral view. Needle was not crossing the neural foramina. Needle 0.5 ml radiocontrast was injected.

Sensory stimulation was performed at 50Hz, patient's pain was reproduced at 0.5 V. On motor stimulation up to 2 volts, there was no motor stimulation of lower extremity. 0.5 ml of 1% Lignocaine was then injected slowly at each level. After waiting 30-60 seconds, ablation was performed utilizing a radiofrequency generator at 80⁰C for 90 seconds. The needles were then withdrawn by 5mm and rotated 180⁰. Then a second ablation was done at 80⁰C for another 90 seconds. After the ablation, the above injectate was given at each level as the needle was removed. Needles were removed intact. A sterile dressing was applied. Similar procedure was carried out at other levels.

The procedure was completed without complications and was tolerated well. After the procedure, the patient was monitored for 30 minutes in the recovery room. The patient (or responsible adult) was given post-procedure and discharge instructions to follow at home. The patient was discharged in stable condition after making a follow-up appointment.

Pre-procedure pain score: _____

Post-procedure pain score: _____

CHAPTER 15

SACROILIAC JOINT INJECTION UNDER FLUOROSCOPY GUIDANCE

Name: _____ age/sex _____date/time _____

PROCEDURE: Fluoroscopy guided Sacroiliac joint injection, left/right side

DIAGNOSIS: _____

PHYSICIAN: _____

MEDICATIONS INJECTED: 0.5 ml of 0.125% Bupivacaine with 20 mg Methylprednisolone/ Triamcinolone

SEDATION MEDICATIONS: None

ANAESTHESIA: Local/sedation/TIVA/General Anesthesia

COMPLICATIONS: None

TECHNIQUE: After confirming written informed consent and NPO status, multipara monitor was attached to the patient. Intravenous access was secured. Time-out was taken to identify the correct patient, procedure and side prior to starting the procedure.

With the patient lying in prone position with pillow under the abdomen at the level of the iliac crests, parts were prepped and draped in the usual sterile fashion using betadine-spirit and sterile fenestrated drape. L5 level, Sacroiliac joint, medial aspect of ipsilateral hip joint was identified on PA view. L5 lower endplate was squared by rotating the image intensifier caudally. C-arm was moved contralateral oblique till anterior and posterior sacroiliac joints were overlapped and crisp lower 1/3rd joint space was seen. Entry point was marked 2 cm from inferior most part of SIJ. Local anesthetic 5 ml of 1% Lignocaine was given by raising a skin wheal and along path of Quincke needle using a 26-gauge 1.25-inch needle.

A 3.5-inch 23-gauge curved tip Quincke needle was advanced 1-2 cm from inferior most part of Sacroiliac joint. Needle was advanced in tunnel view till it hit medial border of Sacroiliac joint. Then it was walked off. A distinct popping sensation was felt once the needle reached the joint.

Needle was confirmed to be 2 cm beyond posterior border of sacrum in lateral view. AP view and 5^0 oblique tilt on each side also confirmed that the needle was in the joint space. After a negative aspirate to make sure that there was no intravascular placement, 0.5 ml Omnipaque 240 contrast was injected, which outlined the Sacroiliac joint with no vascular runoff. After a negative aspiration, the medication was then injected. Needle was removed intact. A sterile dressing was applied.

The procedure was completed without complications and was tolerated well. After the procedure, the patient was monitored for 30 minutes in the recovery room. The patient (or responsible adult) was given post-procedure and discharge instructions to follow at home. The patient was discharged in stable condition after making a follow-up appointment.

Pre-procedure pain score: _____

Post-procedure pain score: _____

Note: Patient was instructed to maintain a pain diary after the block. The patient was also instructed to do the activities that would normally worsen the pain. He/she was asked to note percentage of pain relief obtained at rest and after activity and also duration of pain relief.

CHAPTER 16

RADIOFREQUENCY ABLATION OF SACRAL LATERAL BRANCHES

Name: _____ age/sex _____date/time _____

PROCEDURE: Radiofrequency ablation of sacral lateral branches, left/right side

DIAGNOSIS: _____

PHYSICIAN: _____

MEDICATIONS INJECTED: 0.5 ml of 0.125% Bupivacaine with 20 mg Methylprednisolone/ Triamcinolone

SEDATION MEDICATIONS: Midazolam 1.5 mg, Fentanyl 100mcg IV

ANAESTHESIA: Local/sedation/TIVA/General Anesthesia

COMPLICATIONS: None

TECHNIQUE: After confirming written informed consent and NPO status, multipara monitor was attached to the patient. Intravenous access was secured. Time-out was taken to identify the correct patient, procedure and side prior to starting the procedure.

With the patient lying in prone position with pillow under the abdomen at the level of the iliac crests, parts were prepped and draped in the usual sterile fashion using betadine-spirit and sterile fenestrated drape. L5 vertebra and Sacroiliac joint were identified on PA view. L5 lower endplate was squared. C-arm was moved contralateral oblique to identify first three sacral foramina. Entry points were marked 5-7 mm lateral to posterior foraminal opening to cover areas between 1'O clock to and 5'O clock on right side and from 11'O clock to and 7'O clock on left side. Three entry points were marked at S1 and S2 level and two at S3 level. Entry point at each level were 1-1.5 cm apart from each other. Local anesthetic 5 ml of 1% Lignocaine was given by raising a skin wheal and along path of radiofrequency needle using a 23-gauge 10cm spinal needle.

18 G 100mm long radiofrequency needle with 10mm active tip was inserted at the entry point and advanced till it made bony contact lateral to sacral foramen and medial to sacroiliac joint on AP view. Needle tip was posterior to posterior sacral plate in lateral view. After confirming correct position of needle tip on fluoroscopy, radiofrequency probe was inserted. After positive sensory and negative motor stimulation, treatment medication was given. After waiting for 30-60 seconds, lesioning was done using Cooled RF at 60⁰C for 150 seconds. Similar procedure was repeated at other entry points. One lesion was performed at L5 dorsal rami level, and three at S1 and S2 level and two at S3 level. Lesions were performed at least 5-7 mm lateral to lateral foraminal opening to cover areas between 1'O clock to and 5'O clock on right side and from 11'O clock to and 7'O clock on left side.

The procedure was completed without complications and was tolerated well. After the procedure, the patient was monitored for 30 minutes in the recovery room. The patient (or responsible adult) was given post-procedure and discharge instructions to follow at home. The patient was discharged in stable condition after making a follow-up appointment.

Pre-procedure pain score: _____

Post-procedure pain score: _____

CHAPTER 17

PIRIFORMIS MUSCLE INJECTION

Name: _____ age/sex _____date/time _____

PROCEDURE: Fluoroscopy and nerve stimulator guided piriformis muscle injection, left/right side

DIAGNOSIS: _____

PHYSICIAN: _____

MEDICATIONS INJECTED: 4 ml of 0.5% Bupivacaine with 40 mg Methylprednisolone/ Triamcinolone

SEDATION MEDICATIONS: None

ANAESTHESIA: Local/sedation/TIVA/General Anesthesia

COMPLICATIONS: None

TECHNIQUE: After confirming written informed consent and NPO status, multipara monitor was attached to the patient. Intravenous access was secured. Time-out was taken to identify the correct patient, procedure and side prior to starting the procedure.

With the patient lying in the prone position, the parts were prepped and draped in the usual sterile fashion using betadine-spirit and sterile fenestrated drape. Inferior part of sacroiliac joint was adjusted in the middle of screen on AP view in fluoroscopy. Entry point is marked at the midpoint of line joining greater trochanter and lateral border of sacrum was marked/ point at medial 2/3rd and lateral 1/3rd of the line joining the inferior most part of sacroiliac joint and supero-lateral aspect of acetabulum. Local anesthetic 5 ml of 1% Lignocaine was given at the site by raising a skin wheal and along path of Stimuplex needle using a 26-gauge 1.25-inch needle.

22-gauge Stimuplex needle was introduced perpendicular to skin at entry point. Gluteus maximus contraction was seen at 1.5 mA, 2 Hz. Output was reduced till moderate gluteal twitch seen. Gluteus twitch markedly diminished as the needle was advanced. The needle was advanced till twitching was seen only at the needle hub (dancing needle) which identified piriformis muscle. There was no twitching of leg (sciatic). Rubbery sensation was felt on piercing the muscle.

2 ml of Omnipaque 240 was then injected, which showed diagonal spread from cephalad to caudad towards femoral attachment confirming intramuscular placement. After a negative aspiration, the medication was then injected. Needle was removed intact. A sterile dressing was applied.

The procedure was completed without complications and was tolerated well. After the procedure, the patient was monitored for 30 minutes in the recovery room. Neurological evaluation of the lower limb was done before discharge and found normal. The patient (or responsible adult) was given post-procedure and discharge instructions to follow at home. The patient was discharged in stable condition after making a follow-up appointment.

Pre-procedure pain score: _____

Post-procedure pain score: _____

SECTION 3
KNEE

CHAPTER 1

KNEE INJECTION: ANTEROLATERAL APPROACH

Name: _____ age/sex _____ date/time _____

PROCEDURE: Knee injection using Anterolateral approach under Fluoroscopic guidance, left/right side

DIAGNOSIS: _____

PHYSICIAN: _____

MEDICATIONS INJECTED: 1 ml of Triamcinolone/Methylprednisolone (40 mg) and 4 ml of 1% Lignocaine or 0.25% Bupivacaine / 6 ml Synvisc on each side/6 ml PRP

SEDATION MEDICATIONS: None

ANAESTHESIA: Local/sedation/TIVA/General Anesthesia

COMPLICATIONS: None

TECHNIQUE: After confirming written informed consent, multipara monitor was attached to the patient. Time-out was taken to identify the correct patient, procedure and side prior to starting the procedure.

Patient was positioned supine with hip and knee flexed at 90^0. Parts were prepped and draped in the usual sterile fashion using betadine-spirit and sterile fenestrated drape. Medial and lateral tibial plateau, patellar ligament and tibial tuberosity was palpated. Entry point was marked 1 fingertip above the lateral tibial plateau and 1 fingertip lateral to patellar ligament. 2% Lignocaine was infiltrated in skin, subcutaneous tissue up-to joint capsule using 25-gauge needle.

A 22-gauge 2-inch needle was inserted at the entry point with bevel facing upwards. Needle was advanced at 45^0 from anterior knee surface, towards the intercondylar notch in standard technique/ under the patellar tendon medially towards medial femoral condyle in modified approach. A give way was felt as needle crossed the joint capsule. Aspiration was attempted to rule out vascular placement and remove excess synovial fluid. 2 ml Omnipaque 240 was then injected. On the A-P view, contrast was seen spreading to both sides of the joint (Moustache sign). On lateral fluoroscopy view, contrast was seen spreading into the suprapatellar bursa. Thus, confirming intraarticular placement of the needle. Medication was then injected slowly; it could be injected freely.

The procedure was completed without complications and was tolerated well. After the procedure, the patient was monitored for 30 minutes in the recovery room. The patient (or responsible adult) was given post-procedure and discharge instructions to follow at home. The patient was discharged in stable condition after making a follow-up appointment.

Pre-procedure pain score: _____

Post-procedure pain score: _____

CHAPTER 2

KNEE INJECTION: ANTEROMEDIAL APPROACH

Name: _____ age/sex _____ date/time _____

PROCEDURE: Knee injection using Anteromedial approach under Fluoroscopic guidance, left/right side

DIAGNOSIS: _____

PHYSICIAN: _____

MEDICATIONS INJECTED: 1 ml of Methylprednisolone/Triamcinolone (40 mg) and 4 ml of 1% Lignocaine / 6 ml Synvisc on each side/6 ml PRP

SEDATION MEDICATIONS: None

ANAESTHESIA: Local/sedation/TIVA/General Anesthesia

COMPLICATIONS: None

TECHNIQUE: After confirming written informed consent, multipara monitor was attached to the patient. Time-out was taken to identify the correct patient, procedure and side prior to starting the procedure.

Patient was positioned supine with hip and knee flexed at 90^0. Parts were prepped and draped in the usual sterile fashion using betadine-spirit and sterile fenestrated drape. Medial and lateral tibial plateau, patellar ligament and tibial tuberosity was palpated. Entry point was marked 1 fingertip above the medial tibial plateau and 1 fingertip medial to patellar ligament. 2% Lignocaine was infiltrated in skin, subcutaneous tissue up-to joint capsule using 25-gauge needle.

A 22-gauge 2-inch needle was inserted at the entry point with bevel facing upwards. Needle was advanced at 45^0 from anterior knee surface, towards the intercondylar notch in standard technique/ under the patellar tendon laterally towards lateral femoral condyle in modified approach. A give way was felt as needle crossed the joint capsule. Aspiration was attempted to rule out vascular placement and remove excess synovial fluid. 2 ml Omnipaque 240 was then injected. On the A-P view, contrast was seen spreading to both sides of the joint (Moustache sign). On lateral fluoroscopy view, contrast was seen spreading into the suprapatellar bursa. Thus, confirming intraarticular placement of the needle. Medication was then injected slowly; it could be injected freely.

The procedure was completed without complications and was tolerated well. After the procedure, the patient was monitored for 30 minutes in the recovery room. The patient (or responsible adult) was given post-procedure and discharge instructions to follow at home. The patient was discharged in stable condition after making a follow-up appointment.

Pre-procedure pain score: _____

Post-procedure pain score: _____

CHAPTER 3

KNEE INJECTION: LATERAL
RETROPATELLAR APPROACH

Name: _____ age/sex _____ date/time _____

PROCEDURE: Knee injection Lateral retropatellar approach under Fluoroscopic guidance, left/right side

DIAGNOSIS: _____

PHYSICIAN: _____

MEDICATIONS INJECTED: 1 ml of Methylprednisolone/Triamcinolone (40 mg) and 4 ml of 1% Lignocaine / 6 ml Synvisc on each side/6 ml PRP

SEDATION MEDICATIONS: None

ANAESTHESIA: Local/sedation/TIVA/General Anesthesia

COMPLICATIONS: None

TECHNIQUE: After confirming written informed consent, multipara monitor was attached to the patient. Time-out was taken to identify the correct patient, procedure and side prior to starting the procedure.

Patient was positioned supine with knee extended and elevated using a rolled towel under knee. Parts were prepped and draped in the usual sterile fashion using betadine-spirit and sterile fenestrated drape. Knee joint was visualized in AP view.

Superior and inferior pole of patella was identified. Patella was pushed from medial side to open the lateral space. A groove is palpated underneath the patella on lateral side. Entry point was marked at the junction of upper and middle thirds of patella in the deepest part of lateral retro patellar groove. 2% Lignocaine was infiltrated in skin, subcutaneous tissue up-to joint capsule using 25-gauge needle.

Pressure was applied on the patella medially to tilt it laterally and open the joint space. A 22-gauge 1.5-inch needle was inserted at the entry point and advanced medially and slightly inferiorly with syringe held horizontally. A give way was felt as needle crossed the joint capsule. Aspiration was attempted to rule out vascular placement and remove excess synovial fluid. 2 ml Omnipaque 240 was then injected. On the A-P view, contrast was seen spreading to both sides of the joint (Moustache sign). On lateral fluoroscopy view, contrast was seen spreading into the suprapatellar bursa. Thus, confirming intraarticular placement of the needle. Medication was then injected slowly; it could be injected freely.

The procedure was completed without complications and was tolerated well. After the procedure, the patient was monitored for 30 minutes in the recovery room. The patient (or responsible adult) was given post-procedure and discharge instructions to follow at home. The patient was discharged in stable condition after making a follow-up appointment.

Pre-procedure pain score: _____

Post-procedure pain score: _____

CHAPTER 4

KNEE INJECTION: MEDIAL RETROPATELLAR APPROACH

Name: _____ age/sex _____ date/time _____

PROCEDURE: Knee injection medial retropatellar approach under Fluoroscopic guidance, left/right side

DIAGNOSIS: _____

PHYSICIAN: _____

MEDICATIONS INJECTED: 1 ml of Methylprednisolone/Triamcinolone (40 mg) and 4 ml of 1% Lignocaine / 6 ml Synvisc on each side/6 ml PRP

SEDATION MEDICATIONS: None

ANAESTHESIA: Local/sedation/TIVA/General Anesthesia

COMPLICATIONS: None

TECHNIQUE: After confirming written informed consent, multipara monitor was attached to the patient. Time-out was taken to identify the correct patient, procedure and side prior to starting the procedure.

Patient was positioned supine with knee extended and elevated using a rolled towel under knee. Parts were prepped and draped in the usual sterile fashion using betadine-spirit and sterile fenestrated drape. Knee joint was visualized in AP view.

Superior and inferior pole of patella was identified. Patella was pushed from lateral side to open the medial space. A groove is palpated underneath the patella on medial side. Entry point was marked halfway between the poles in the deepest part of medial parapatellar groove. 2% Lignocaine was infiltrated in skin, subcutaneous tissue up-to joint capsule using 25-gauge needle.

Pressure was applied on the patella laterally to tilt it medially and open the joint space. A 22-gauge 1.5-inch needle was inserted at the entry point and advanced laterally with syringe held horizontally. A give way was felt as needle crossed the joint capsule. Aspiration was attempted to rule out vascular placement and remove excess synovial fluid. 2 ml Omnipaque 240 was then injected. On the A-P view, contrast was seen spreading to both sides of the joint (Moustache sign). On lateral fluoroscopy view, contrast was seen spreading into the suprapatellar bursa. Thus, confirming intraarticular placement of the needle. Medication was then injected slowly; it could be injected freely.

The procedure was completed without complications and was tolerated well. After the procedure, the patient was monitored for 30 minutes in the recovery room. The patient (or responsible adult) was given post-procedure and discharge instructions to follow at home. The patient was discharged in stable condition after making a follow-up appointment.

Pre-procedure pain score: _____

Post-procedure pain score: _____

CHAPTER 5

KNEE INJECTION: SUPEROLATERAL APPROACH

Name: _____ age/sex _____ date/time _____

PROCEDURE: Knee injection Superolateral approach under Fluoroscopic guidance, left/right side

DIAGNOSIS: _____

PHYSICIAN: _____

MEDICATIONS INJECTED: 1 ml (40 mg) of Methylprednisolone/Triamcinolone and 4 ml of 1% Lignocaine / 6 ml Synvisc on each side/6 ml PRP

SEDATION MEDICATIONS: None

ANAESTHESIA: Local/sedation/TIVA/General Anesthesia

COMPLICATIONS: None

TECHNIQUE: After confirming written informed consent, multipara monitor was attached to the patient. Time-out was taken to identify the correct patient, procedure and side prior to starting the procedure.

Patient was positioned supine with knee extended and elevated using a rolled towel under knee. Parts were prepped and draped in the usual sterile fashion using betadine-spirit and sterile fenestrated drape. Knee joint was visualized in AP view.

Superior and lateral border of patella was palpated. Entry point was marked at the intersection of imaginary lines joining horizontal line from superior border of patella and another line from lateral border of patella. 2% Lignocaine was infiltrated in skin, subcutaneous tissue up-to joint capsule using 25-gauge needle.

A 22-gauge 1.5-inch needle was inserted at the entry point and advanced medially, aiming at anterior femoral cortex. A give way was felt as needle crossed the joint capsule. Aspiration was attempted to rule out vascular placement and remove excess synovial fluid. 2 ml Omnipaque 240 was then injected. On the A-P view, contrast was seen spreading to both sides of the joint (Moustache sign). On lateral fluoroscopy view, contrast was seen spreading into the suprapatellar bursa. Thus, confirming intraarticular placement of the needle. Medication was then injected slowly; it could be injected freely.

The procedure was completed without complications and was tolerated well. After the procedure, the patient was monitored for 30 minutes in the recovery room. The patient (or responsible adult) was given post-procedure and discharge instructions to follow at home. The patient was discharged in stable condition after making a follow-up appointment.

Pre-procedure pain score: _____

Post-procedure pain score: _____

CHAPTER 6

DIAGNOSTIC GENICULAR NERVE BLOCK

Name: _____ age/sex _____ date/time _____

PROCEDURE: Diagnostic genicular nerve block under Fluoroscopic guidance left/right side

DIAGNOSIS: _____

PHYSICIAN: _____

MEDICATIONS INJECTED: 1 ml of 2% Lignocaine at each site

SEDATION MEDICATIONS: None

ANESTHESIA: Local/sedation/TIVA/General Anesthesia

COMPLICATIONS: None

TECHNIQUE: After confirming written informed consent and NPO status, multipara monitor was attached to the patient. Intravenous access was secured. Time-out was taken to identify the correct patient, procedure and side prior to starting the procedure.

Patient was positioned supine with knee extended and elevated using a rolled towel under knee. Parts were prepped and draped in the usual sterile fashion using betadine-spirit and sterile fenestrated drape. AP view of distal femur and proximal tibia was obtained on fluoroscopy. Four target sites were identified. First at the junction of the femoral diaphysis and the medial femoral epicondyle, second at the junction of femoral diaphysis and the lateral femoral epicondyle, 3rd at the junction of tibial diaphysis and medial tibial condyle and fourth one at 2 cm cephalad to upper patellar border. Local anesthetic 2 ml of 1% Lignocaine was given at each site by raising a skin wheal and along path of spinal needle using a 26-gauge 1.25-inch needle.

In an A-P fluoroscopic view, 23-gauge curved tip spinal needles were introduced through the anesthetized skin at the four entry points. Needles were advanced in tunnel view. Placement of needles was confirmed to be halfway across the thickness of femur at first two entry points and halfway across tibia for third entry point in lateral fluoroscopic view. After a negative aspirate to make sure that there was no intravascular placement 1 ml of non-ionic contrast was injected in real time fluoroscopy which showed no vascular uptake. Then, 1 ml of the 2% Lignocaine was injected slowly at each site. Needles were all removed intact. A sterile dressing was applied.

The procedure was completed without complications and was tolerated well. After the procedure, the patient was monitored for 30 minutes in the recovery room. The patient (or responsible adult) was given post-procedure and discharge instructions to follow at home. The patient was discharged in stable condition after making a follow-up appointment.

Pre-procedure pain score: _____

Post-procedure pain score: _____

Note: Patient was instructed to maintain a pain diary after the block. The patient was also instructed to do the activities that would normally worsen the pain. He/she was asked to note percentage of pain relief obtained at rest and after activity and also duration of pain relief.

CHAPTER 7

GENICULAR NERVE RADIOFREQUENCY ABLATION

Name: _____ age/sex _____ date/time _____

PROCEDURE: Radiofrequency Ablation of genicular nerve under Fluoroscopic guidance left/right side

DIAGNOSIS:

PHYSICIAN: _____

MEDICATIONS INJECTED: 1 ml of 2% Lignocaine at each site

SEDATION MEDICATIONS: None

ANAESTHESIA: Local/sedation/TIVA/General Anesthesia

COMPLICATIONS: None

TECHNIQUE: After confirming written informed consent and NPO status, multipara monitor was attached to the patient. Intravenous access was secured. Time-out was taken to identify the correct patient, procedure and side prior to starting the procedure.

Patient was positioned supine with knee extended and elevated using a rolled towel under knee. Parts were prepped and draped in the usual sterile fashion using betadine-spirit and sterile fenestrated drape. AP view of distal femur and proximal tibia was obtained on fluoroscopy. Four target sites were identified. First at the junction of the femoral diaphysis and the medial femoral epicondyle, second at the junction of femoral diaphysis and the lateral femoral epicondyle, 3rd at the junction of tibial diaphysis and medial tibial condyle and fourth one at 2 cm cephalad to upper patellar border. Local anesthetic 2 ml of 1% Lignocaine was given at each site by raising a skin wheal and along path of RF needle using a 26-gauge 1.25-inch needle.

In an A-P fluoroscopic view, 18G curved RF needle with a 10 mm active tip was introduced through the anesthetized skin, at the four entry points. Needles were advanced in tunnel view. Placement of needles was confirmed to be halfway across the thickness of femur at first two entry points and halfway across tibia for third entry point in lateral fluoroscopic view. Stylet was removed. After a negative aspirate to make sure that there was no intravascular placement 1 ml of non-ionic contrast was injected in real time fluoroscopy to which showed no vascular uptake. Radiofrequency probes were inserted. Motor stimulation was done with 2Hz up to 1V to rule out any lower extremity motor activity. Then, 1 ml of the 2% Lignocaine was injected slowly at each site after removing the probe. Cooled RF was used to ablate the nerves at 60°C for 2.5 minutes. The needle was then withdrawn about 5mm and a second ablation was done with the same settings. Similar lesioning was done at each site. All the needles were removed intact. A sterile dressing was applied.

The procedure was completed without complications and was tolerated well. After the procedure, the patient was monitored for 2 hours in the recovery room. The patient (or responsible adult) was given post-procedure and discharge instructions to follow at home. The patient was discharged in stable condition after making a follow-up appointment.

Pre-procedure pain score: _____

Post-procedure pain score: _____

SECTION 4
HIP

CHAPTER 1

HIP INJECTION: LATERAL APPROACH

Name: _____ age/sex _____date/time _____

PROCEDURE: Hip injection lateral approach under Fluoroscopic guidance, left/right side

DIAGNOSIS: _____

PHYSICIAN: _____

MEDICATIONS INJECTED: 1 ml of Triamcinolone/Methylprednisolone (40 mg) and 4 ml of 1% Lignocaine/0.25% Bupivacaine

SEDATION MEDICATIONS: None

ANAESTHESIA: Local/sedation/TIVA/General Anesthesia

COMPLICATIONS: None

TECHNIQUE: After confirming written informed consent, multipara monitor was attached to the patient. Time-out was taken to identify the correct patient, procedure and side prior to starting the procedure.

Patient was positioned lying in the supine with knee extended and foot slightly internal rotated. Parts were prepped and draped in the usual sterile fashion using betadine-spirit and sterile fenestrated drape. Hip joint and Greater trochanter of femur was visualized in AP view. Entry point was marked 1cm above greater trochanter. 2% Lignocaine was infiltrated in skin, subcutaneous tissue using 25-gauge needle.

23-gauge spinal needle was inserted perpendicular to skin, parallel to floor, 1cm above Greater trochanter of femur. Needle was advanced medially under intermittent fluoroscopy until the femoral neck was reached. Aspiration was attempted rule out vascular placement and remove excess synovial fluid. 1 ml Omnipaque 240 was then injected. Contrast was seen inside capsule lining femoral head on AP view thus confirming intraarticular spread. There was no vascular spread. Medication was then injected slowly; it could be injected freely. Needle was removed intact. Sterile dressing was applied.

The procedure was completed without complications and was tolerated well. After the procedure, the patient was monitored for 30 minutes in the recovery room. The patient (or responsible adult) was given post-procedure and discharge instructions to follow at home. The patient was discharged in stable condition after making a follow-up appointment.

Pre-procedure pain score: _____

Post-procedure pain score: _____

CHAPTER 2

HIP INJECTION: ANTERIOR APPROACH

Name: _____ age/sex _____ date/time _____

PROCEDURE: Hip injection anterior approach under Fluoroscopic guidance, left/right side

DIAGNOSIS: _____

PHYSICIAN: _____

MEDICATIONS INJECTED: 1 ml of Triamcinolone/Methylprednisolone (40 mg) and 4 ml of 1% Lignocaine/0.25% Bupivacaine

SEDATION MEDICATIONS: None

ANAESTHESIA: Local/sedation/TIVA/General Anesthesia

COMPLICATIONS: None

TECHNIQUE: After confirming written informed consent, multipara monitor was attached to the patient. Time-out was taken to identify the correct patient, procedure and side prior to starting the procedure.

Patient was positioned lying in the supine with knee extended and foot slightly internal rotated. Parts were prepped and draped in the usual sterile fashion using betadine-spirit and sterile fenestrated drape. Hip joint and neck of femur was visualized in AP view. Entry point was marked at the neck of femur on AP view. 2% Lignocaine was infiltrated in skin, subcutaneous tissue using 25-gauge needle.

Femoral artery was palpated. 23-gauge spinal needle was inserted perpendicular to skin, at the entry point i.e., neck of femur. Needle was advanced vertically down in tunnel view under intermittent fluoroscopy until the femoral neck was reached. Aspiration was attempted rule out vascular placement and remove excess synovial fluid. 1 ml Omnipaque 240 was then injected. Contrast was seen inside capsule lining femoral head on AP view thus confirming intraarticular spread. There was no vascular spread. Medication was then injected slowly; it could be injected freely. Needle was removed intact. Sterile dressing was applied.

The procedure was completed without complications and was tolerated well. After the procedure, the patient was monitored for 30 minutes in the recovery room. The patient (or responsible adult) was given post-procedure and discharge instructions to follow at home. The patient was discharged in stable condition after making a follow-up appointment.

Pre-procedure pain score: _____

Post-procedure pain score: _____

SECTION 5
ABDOMEN AND PELVIS

CHAPTER 1

CELIAC PLEXUS BLOCK

Name: _____ age/sex _____ date/time _____

PROCEDURE: Celiac plexus block under fluoroscopy guidance, Bilateral/ left/ right side

DIAGNOSIS: _____

PHYSICIAN: _____

MEDICATIONS INJECTED: 20 ml 0.5% Bupivacaine on each side

SEDATION MEDICATIONS: None

ANAESTHESIA: Local/sedation/TIVA/General Anesthesia

COMPLICATIONS: None

TECHNIQUE: Preoperatively, patient received intravenous 1000 ml RL over 8 hours.

After confirming written informed consent and NPO status, multipara monitor was attached to the patient. Intravenous access was secured. Time-out was taken to identify the correct patient, procedure and side prior to starting the procedure.

With the patient lying in the prone position, the parts were prepped and draped in the usual sterile fashion using betadine-spirit and sterile fenestrated drape. In AP view, L1 level vertebral body was identified and superior endplate was squared. Then C-arm intensifier was then turned ipsilateral oblique until 2/3rd of the L1 transverse process was under the L1 vertebral body. Entry point was marked at the lateral border of vertebral body just below the transverse process. Local anesthetic 5 ml of 1% Lignocaine was given at the entry point by raising a skin wheal and going down to the hub of the 26-gauge 1.25-inch needle.

A 23-gauge 15 cm spinal needle with curved tip was inserted at the entry point. It was advanced in tunnel view under intermittent fluoroscopy, till it reached the anterolateral margin of L1 vertebral body. With a lateral fluoroscopic view, the needle was advanced about 2 cm anterior to the L1 vertebral body. In AP view, needle was seen in lower 1/3rd of T12 vertebral body or upper 1/3rd of L1 vertebral body.

While aspirating during advancement of the needle, the aorta was expectedly entered and the needle slowly advanced in small increments until negative aspiration. 4 ml of Omnipaque 240 contrast was injected. In the AP view, the contrast dye is seen in the midline and concentrated around vertebral bodies T12 and L1. It did not spread beyond the contours of the vertebral bodies. Vacuole-like brightening appearance was seen confirming correct placement of needle tip. In lateral view, a smooth contour was seen in front of vertebral bodies. There was no vascular uptake and no dye spread dorsally in the direction of nerve roots. Then medication was injected slowly in 5 ml increments, aspirating each time to confirm that the needle is not slipped back into the aorta. Similar technique was then repeated for the opposite side. Needles were removed intact. A sterile dressing was applied.

The procedure was completed without complications and was tolerated well. After the procedure, the patient was monitored for 2 hours in the recovery room. The patient (or responsible adult) was given post-procedure and discharge instructions to follow at home. The patient was discharged in stable condition after making a follow-up appointment.

Pre-procedure pain score: _____

Post-procedure pain score: _____

Note: For chemical neurolysis in malignant pain: If there was no neurologic deficits 10 min after injection of local anesthetic, 10 ml of neurolytic agent (absolute alcohol) was injected on each side.

Close hemodynamic and neurological monitoring was done overnight.

Patient was kept well-hydrated.

CHAPTER 2

SPLANCHNIC NERVE BLOCK

Name: _____ age/sex _____ date/time _____

PROCEDURE: Splanchnic nerve block under fluoroscopy guidance, left/right side

DIAGNOSIS: _____

PHYSICIAN: _____

MEDICATIONS INJECTED: 12 ml 0.25% Bupivacaine on each side

SEDATION MEDICATIONS: Midazolam (1.5mg)

ANAESTHESIA: Local/sedation/TIVA/General Anesthesia

COMPLICATIONS: None

TECHNIQUE:

Patient received 500 ml RL prior to procedure, IV antibiotic 30 minutes prior and Midazolam (1.5mg) for sedation.

After confirming written informed consent and NPO status, multipara monitor was attached to the patient. Time-out was taken to identify the correct patient, procedure and side prior to starting the procedure.

With the patient lying in the prone position, the parts were prepped and draped in the usual sterile fashion using betadine-spirit and sterile fenestrated drape.

The anatomical target site was determined using fluoroscopy by squaring off the superior endplate of T12, ipsilaterally obliquing the image intensifier until the tip of the T12 transverse process was at the anterolateral border of the T12 vertebral body. Entry point was marked below head of 11th rib, at the costovertebral junction, below transverse process along the lateral border of vertebral body. Local anesthetic 5 ml of 1% Lignocaine was given by raising a skin wheal and going down to the hub of the 26-gauge 1.25-inch needle.

A 20-gauge 15 cm Quincke needle was inserted at the entry point. Needle was directed medially, towards T12 vertebral body, in tunnel view till bony contact was made with the T12 vertebral body then needle was rotated to keep curve lateral. Grating sensation may be felt as needle moves along T12 vertebral body. Needle was advanced using intermittent fluoroscopy. After confirming needle position at the junction of ant 1/3 and post 2/3 of vertebral body on lateral view, and needle not crossing facet line and mid-pedicular line in AP view, 2 ml of Omnipaque 240 contrast was injected. In AP view, contrast was seen spreading unilaterally in linear pattern, along the anterolateral surface of the T11-T12 vertebral body, with no vascular uptake. Similar technique was then repeated for the opposite side with contrast injected again to show unilateral spread along anterolateral T11-T12 vertebral body. Medication was then injected slowly in 3 ml increments after negative aspirations. Needles were removed intact. A sterile dressing was applied.

The procedure was completed without complications and was tolerated well. After the procedure, the patient was monitored closely for 2 hours in the recovery room. Hemodynamic and neurologic monitoring was done. Patient was watched for hypotension and diarrhea. Xray chest was done after 2 hours to r/o pneumothorax. Patient (or responsible adult) was given post-procedure and discharge instructions to follow at home. The patient was discharged in stable condition after making a follow-up appointment.

Pre-procedure pain score: _____

Post-procedure pain score: _____

Note: For Chemical neurolysis, initially 2 ml 1% Lignocaine was given to avoid burning pain and then 10 ml alcohol mixed with 2 ml contrast was given to visualize spread. Needle was flushed with 1 ml saline prior to and while removing needle to avoid spillage in the track.

CHAPTER 3

DIAGNOSTIC LUMBAR SYMPATHETIC BLOCK

Name: _____ age/sex _____ date/time _____

PROCEDURE: Lumbar sympathetic block under Fluoroscopic guidance, left/right side

DIAGNOSIS: _____

PHYSICIAN: _____

MEDICATIONS INJECTED: 15 ml 0.25% Bupivacaine

SEDATION MEDICATIONS: None

ANAESTHESIA: Local/sedation/TIVA/General Anesthesia

COMPLICATIONS: None

TECHNIQUE: After confirming written informed consent and NPO status, multipara monitor was attached to the patient. Surface thermometry probe was attached on both the lower extremities. Intravenous access was secured. Time-out was taken to identify the correct patient, procedure and side prior to starting the procedure.

With the patient lying in the prone position with pillow under abdomen, parts were prepped and draped in the usual sterile fashion using betadine-spirit and sterile fenestrated drape.

The anatomical target site was determined using fluoroscopy by squaring off the superior endplate of L2, and then ipsilaterally obliquing the C-arm intensifier until the tip of L2 transverse process was in line with lateral border of the L2 vertebral body. Entry point was marked at lateral border of L2 vertebral body, just above the transverse process. Local anesthetic was given by raising a skin wheal and going down to the hub of the 27-gauge 1.25-inch needle.

A 22-gauge Chiba needle was inserted at the entry point with curve medially. Needle was advanced in tunnel view till bony contact was made with the L2 vertebral body then needle was rotated to keep curve lateral. It was advanced further till the needle tip was at the anterior border of vertebral body, at the junction of the upper two thirds, lower one third of the vertebral body in lateral view but not crossing mid-pedicular line on AP view. Then 2 ml Omnipaque 240 contrast was injected. It was seen along the anterior border of vertebral column on lateral view and vacuolated appearance was seen in AP view with no vascular uptake. Needle aspiration was performed and medication was then injected slowly. Similar procedure was repeated at L3 and L4 levels. Needles were removed intact. A sterile dressing was applied.

The procedure was completed without complications and was tolerated well. After the procedure, the patient was monitored for 2 hours in the recovery room. Monitoring was done for hemodynamic stability, Skin temperature, Sensory/ motor function of lower extremity, Vasodilation, change of color, decreased sweating, and pain reduction. The patient (or responsible adult) was given post-procedure and discharge instructions to follow at home. The patient was discharged in stable condition after making a follow-up appointment.

Right lower extremity: Pre-injection skin temp = _____ Post-injection skin temp =_____

Left lower extremity: Pre-injection skin temp = _____ Post-injection skin temp = _____

Pre-procedure pain score: _____

Post-procedure pain score: _____

Note: Patient was instructed to maintain a pain diary after the block. The patient was also instructed to do the activities that would normally worsen the pain. He/she was asked to note percentage of pain relief obtained at rest and after activity and also duration of pain relief.

CHAPTER 4

LUMBAR SYMPATHETIC RADIOFREQUENCY ABLATION

Name: _____ age/sex _____date/time _____

PROCEDURE: Lumbar sympathetic radiofrequency ablation under Fluoroscopic guidance, left/right side

DIAGNOSIS: _____

PHYSICIAN: _____

MEDICATIONS INJECTED: 10 ml 0.25% Bupivacaine

SEDATION MEDICATIONS: None

ANAESTHESIA: Local/sedation/TIVA/General Anesthesia

COMPLICATIONS: None

TECHNIQUE: After confirming written informed consent and NPO status, multipara monitor was attached to the patient. Intravenous access was secured. Time-out was taken to identify the correct patient, procedure and side prior to starting the procedure.

With the patient lying in the prone position, the parts were prepped and draped in the usual sterile fashion using betadine-spirit and sterile fenestrated drape. The anatomical target site was determined using fluoroscopy by squaring off the superior endplate of L2, and then ipsilaterally obliquing the C-arm intensifier until the tip of L2 transverse process was in line with lateral border of the L2 vertebral body. Entry point was marked at lateral border of L2 vertebral body, just above the transverse process. Local anesthetic was given by raising a skin wheal and going down to the hub of the 27-gauge 1.25-inch needle.

22-gauge, 15 cm curved tip RF needle with 10 mm active tip was inserted at entry point with curve medially. Needle was advanced end-on till bony contact was made with the L2 vertebral body then needle was rotated to keep curve lateral. It was advanced further till the needle tip was at the anterior border of vertebral body in lateral view but not crossing mid-pedicular line on AP view. Then 2 ml Omnipaque 240 contrast was injected. It was seen as thin line along the anterior border of vertebral column on lateral view and vacuolated appearance was seen in AP view with no vascular uptake. Needles were placed at L3 and L4 levels in similar manner. Radiofrequency ablation was done at 80^0 C, 2 cycles for 1.30 and 1.00 min at each level after positive sensory stimulation at 50 Hz at _____ V and negative motor stimulation at 2 Hz at 1.2V (there were no limb response). Needles were removed intact. A sterile dressing was applied.

The procedure was completed without complications and was tolerated well. After the procedure, the patient was monitored for 2 hours in the recovery room. Monitoring was done for hemodynamic stability, Skin temperature, Sensory/ motor function of lower extremity, Vasodilation, change of color, decreased sweating, and pain reduction. The patient (or responsible adult) was given post-procedure and discharge instructions to follow at home. The patient was discharged in stable condition after making a follow-up appointment

Right lower extremity: Pre-injection skin temp = _____ Post-injection skin temp =_____

Left lower extremity: Pre-injection skin temp = _____ Post-injection skin temp = _____

Pre-procedure pain score: _____

Post-procedure pain score: _____

CHAPTER 5

SUPERIOR HYPOGASTRIC BLOCK

Name: _____ age/sex _____ date/time _____

PROCEDURE: Superior hypogastric block under fluoroscopy guidance

DIAGNOSIS: _____

PHYSICIAN: _____

MEDICATIONS INJECTED: 15 ml 0.25% Bupivacaine/ 1% Lignocaine on each side

SEDATION MEDICATIONS: Midazolam (1.5mg)

ANAESTHESIA: Local/sedation/TIVA/General Anesthesia

COMPLICATIONS: None

TECHNIQUE:

After confirming written informed consent and NPO status, multipara monitor was attached to the patient. Time-out was taken to identify the correct patient, procedure and side prior to starting the procedure.

With the patient lying in the prone position and pillow under abdomen, parts were prepped and draped in the usual sterile fashion using betadine-spirit and sterile fenestrated drape. The anatomical target site was determined using fluoroscopy by squaring off the superior endplate of L5 and ipsilaterally obliquing the C-arm intensifier until the tip of the L5 transverse process was at the anterolateral border of the L5 vertebral body. Triangle made by iliac crest, Transverse process and vertebral body was identified and marked as needle entry point. Local anesthetic 5 ml of 1% Lignocaine was given by raising a skin wheal and going down to the hub of the 26-gauge 1.25-inch needle.

A 20-gauge 15 cm Quincke needle with curved tip was inserted and was directed medially, towards L5 vertebral body, in tunnel view. Needle was advanced using intermittent fluoroscopy. Grating sensation was felt as needle moves along L5 vertebral body. Needle curve was turned lateral and was advanced. Pop was felt when needle pierced psoas fascia. In lateral view, needle was confirmed to be just anterior to the vertebral body, in inferior one-third of the L5 vertebral body and in AP view, it was in the lateral 1/5th of vertebral body, in front of upper part of sacral promontory, close to lateral border of vertebral body, not crossing mid-pedicular line. Then 2 ml of Omnipaque 240 contrast was injected. Contrast was seen as linear spread in front of vertebral body on lateral view and at the anterolateral border of L5-S1 on AP view with no vascular uptake. Medication was then injected slowly in 3 ml increments after negative aspirations. Procedure is repeated on opposite side. Needles were removed intact. A sterile dressing was applied.

The procedure was completed without complications and was tolerated well. After the procedure, the patient was monitored closely for 4 hours in the recovery room. Hemodynamic and neurologic monitoring was done. Patient (or responsible adult) was given post-procedure and discharge instructions to follow at home. The patient was discharged in stable condition after making a follow-up appointment.

Pre-procedure pain score: _____

Post-procedure pain score: _____

Note: For Chemical neurolysis in malignancy, initially 2 ml 1% Lignocaine was given to avoid burning pain and then 10 ml 50% alcohol mixed with 2 ml contrast was given to visualize spread. Needle was flushed with 1 ml saline prior to and while removing needle to avoid spillage in the track. Patient was advised absolute bed rest without position change, for 4 hours to avoid unwanted spread of neurolytic.

44

CHAPTER 6

GANGLION IMPAR INJECTION: TRANSSACROCOCCYGEAL APPROACH

Name: _____ age/sex _____ date/time _____

PROCEDURE: fluoroscopy guided ganglion impar injection, trans-sacrococcygeal approach

DIAGNOSIS: _____

PHYSICIAN: _____

MEDICATIONS INJECTED: 40 mg Triamcinolone/Methylprednisolone with 4 ml of 1% Lignocaine/ 0.25% Bupivacaine

ANAESTHESIA: Local/sedation/TIVA/General Anesthesia

SEDATION MEDICATIONS: None

COMPLICATIONS: None

TECHNIQUE: After confirming written informed consent and NPO status, multipara monitor was attached to the patient. Intravenous access was secured. Time-out was taken to identify the correct patient, procedure and side prior to starting the procedure.

Patient was positioned prone with pillow under lower abdomen and pelvis. Parts were prepped and draped in the usual sterile fashion using betadine-spirit and sterile fenestrated drape. Sacrum and coccygeal bones were identified in AP view in the midline, sacrococcygeal joint was identified in lateral view of fluoroscopy. Local anesthetic 5 ml of 1% Lignocaine was given at sacrococcygeal disc at superior aspect of intergluteal crease just below sacral hiatus by raising a skin wheal and subcutaneous tissue using a 26-gauge 1.25-inch needle.

A 22-gauge 1.5-inch needle was inserted at the marked site through sacrococcygeal disc under lateral view of fluoroscopy. A 25-gauge Spinal needle was then introduced through the needle to reach the anterior line of coccygeal bone. Then 2 ml Omnipaque 240 was injected. It was seen as 'comma sign' along the anterior aspect of coccygeal bones in the retroperitoneal space on lateral view. On AP view, it was seen in front of the sacrococcygeal junction in midline. There was no vascular runoff. After aspiration, treatment medication was injected. The needle was then retracted back to the sacrococcygeal ligament area. Both the needles were removed. Pressure was applied at the injection site. Sterile dressing was applied.

The procedure was completed without complications and was tolerated well. After the procedure, the patient was monitored for 30 minutes in the recovery room. The patient (or responsible adult) was given post-procedure and discharge instructions to follow at home. The patient was discharged in stable condition after making a follow-up appointment.

Pre-procedure pain score: _____

Post-procedure pain score: _____

CHAPTER 7

GANGLION IMPAR INJECTION: TRANS-COCCYGEAL APPROACH

Name: _____ age/sex _____ date/time _____

PROCEDURE: fluoroscopy guided ganglion impar injection, trans-coccygeal approach

DIAGNOSIS: _____

PHYSICIAN: _____

MEDICATIONS INJECTED: 40 mg Triamcinolone/Methylprednisolone with 4 ml of 1% Lignocaine/ 0.25% Bupivacaine

ANAESTHESIA: Local/sedation/TIVA/General Anesthesia

SEDATION MEDICATIONS: None

COMPLICATIONS: None

TECHNIQUE: After confirming written informed consent and NPO status, multipara monitor was attached to the patient. Intravenous access was secured. Time-out was taken to identify the correct patient, procedure and side prior to starting the procedure.

Patient was positioned prone with pillow under lower abdomen and pelvis. Parts were prepped and draped in the usual sterile fashion using betadine-spirit and sterile fenestrated drape. Sacrum and coccygeal bones were identified in AP view in the midline, intercoccygeal joint was identified in lateral view of fluoroscopy. Local anesthetic 5 ml of 1% Lignocaine was given at first intercoccygeal disc at superior aspect of intergluteal crease by raising a skin wheal and subcutaneous tissue using a 26-gauge 1.25-inch needle.

A22-gauge 1.5-inch needle was inserted at the marked site through trans-coccygeal junction and advanced under lateral fluoroscopy to reach the anterior coccygeal line. Then 2 ml Omnipaque 240 was injected. It was seen as 'reverse comma sign' in the retroperitoneal space on lateral view. On AP view, it's in front of the coccyx in midline. There was no vascular runoff. After aspiration, treatment medication was injected. Needle was removed intact. Pressure was applied at the injection site. Sterile dressing was applied.

The procedure was completed without complications and was tolerated well. After the procedure, the patient was monitored for 30 minutes in the recovery room. The patient (or responsible adult) was given post-procedure and discharge instructions to follow at home. The patient was discharged in stable condition after making a follow-up appointment.

Pre-procedure pain score: _____

Post-procedure pain score: _____

46

CHAPTER 8

ILIOINGUINAL NERVE BLOCK: CLASSICAL APPROACH

Name: _____ age/sex _____date/time _____

PROCEDURE: Landmark guided ilioinguinal nerve block using classic approach, left/right side

DIAGNOSIS: _____

PHYSICIAN: _____

MEDICATIONS INJECTED: total 19 ml of 0.25% Bupivacaine with 1 ml (40 mg) Methylprednisolone/Triamcinolone

SEDATION MEDICATIONS: None

ANAESTHESIA: Local/sedation/TIVA/General Anesthesia

COMPLICATIONS: None

TECHNIQUE: After confirming written informed consent and NPO status, multipara monitor was attached to the patient. Intravenous access was secured. Time-out was taken to identify the correct patient, procedure and side prior to starting the procedure.

With the patient lying in the supine position, the parts were prepped and draped in the usual sterile fashion using betadine-spirit and sterile fenestrated drape.

Anterior Superior Iliac Spine (ASIS) was palpated. Entry point was marked 2 cm medial and 2 cm inferior to ASIS. 22-gauge short bevel Needle was inserted at the entry point perpendicular to the skin. After feeling first pop, 2 ml treatment medication was given after confirming negative aspiration. Then needle was advanced and second pop was felt. Again, 2 ml treatment medication was given after confirming negative aspiration. Needle was retracted up to skin and inserted with 45⁰ angles medially. Again 2 pops were felt and 2 ml treatment medication was injected after each pop after confirming negative aspiration. Needle was retracted up to skin and inserted with 45⁰ angles laterally. Again 2 pops were felt and 2 ml treatment medication was injected after each pop after confirming negative aspiration. Needle was removed intact. A sterile dressing was applied.

The procedure was completed without complications and was tolerated well. After the procedure, the patient was monitored for 30 minutes in the recovery room. Patient was assessed for quadriceps weakness before allowing ambulation. The patient (or responsible adult) was given post-procedure and discharge instructions to follow at home. The patient was discharged in stable condition after making a follow-up appointment.

Pre-procedure pain score: _____

Post-procedure pain score: _____

CHAPTER 9

ILIOINGUINAL NERVE BLOCK: MODIFIED APPROACH

Name: _____ age/sex _____ date/time _____

PROCEDURE: PNL guided ilioinguinal nerve block using modified approach, left/right side

DIAGNOSIS: _____

PHYSICIAN: _____

MEDICATIONS INJECTED: 20 ml of 0.25% Bupivacaine with 1 ml (40 mg) Methylprednisolone/Triamcinolone

SEDATION MEDICATIONS: None

ANAESTHESIA: Local/sedation/TIVA/General Anesthesia

COMPLICATIONS: None

TECHNIQUE: After confirming written informed consent and NPO status, multipara monitor was attached to the patient. Intravenous access was secured. Time-out was taken to identify the correct patient, procedure and side prior to starting the procedure.

With the patient lying in the supine position, the parts were prepped and draped in the usual sterile fashion using betadine-spirit and sterile fenestrated drape.

Anterior Superior Iliac Spine (ASIS) was palpated. Entry point was marked 5 cm posterior and 5 cm superior to ASIS. A 5 cm insulated short bevel Needle was inserted at the entry point perpendicular to the skin. After feeling two pops, contraction of anterior abdominal muscles was seen. Initially current was set at 1.5mA and it was reduced gradually. Needle position was adjusted till evoked motor response was seen at 0.5mA. 20 ml treatment medication was given after confirming negative aspiration. Needle was removed intact. A sterile dressing was applied.

The procedure was completed without complications and was tolerated well. After the procedure, the patient was monitored for 30 minutes in the recovery room. Patient was assessed for quadriceps weakness before allowing ambulation. The patient (or responsible adult) was given post-procedure and discharge instructions to follow at home. The patient was discharged in stable condition after making a follow-up appointment.

Pre-procedure pain score: _____

Post-procedure pain score: _____

SECTION 6
CHEST AND SHOULDER

CHAPTER 1

SUPRASCAPULAR NERVE BLOCK

Name: _____ age/sex _____ date/time _____

PROCEDURE: Suprascapular nerve block, posterior approach, under Fluoroscopic guidance, left/right side

DIAGNOSIS: _____

PHYSICIAN: _____

MEDICATIONS INJECTED: 2 ml 0.25% Bupivacaine with 40 mg Triamcinolone/ Methylprednisolone

SEDATION MEDICATIONS: None

ANAESTHESIA: Local/sedation/TIVA/General Anesthesia

COMPLICATIONS: None

TECHNIQUE: After confirming written informed consent and NPO status, multipara monitor was attached to the patient. Intravenous access was secured. Time-out was taken to identify the correct patient, procedure and side prior to starting the procedure.

Patient was positioned prone with pillow under chest, head slightly flexed and arm positioned at patient's side / arm positioned under head. Parts were prepped and draped in the usual sterile fashion using betadine-spirit and sterile fenestrated drape.

C-arm was rotated craniocaudal till suprascapular notch was identified just medial to base of coracoid process on AP view. Entry point was marked over inferior margin of suprascapular notch. Local anesthetic was given by raising a skin wheal and in subcutaneous tissue with a 25-gauge 1.25-inch needle.

A 22-gauge 10cm spinal needle was advanced in tunnel view until tip contacted scapula at the inferior margin of scapular notch. Then the needle was walked off by withdrawing 1-2mm, redirecting and readvancing.

During the procedure, when paresthesia was elicited, 1 ml of Omnipaque 240 was injected. Contrast was seen suffusing through the suprascapular notch. After aspiration, treatment medication was slowly injected. Needle was removed intact. A sterile dressing was applied.

The procedure was completed without complications and was tolerated well. After the procedure, the patient was monitored closely for 2 hours in the recovery room. Post-procedure X-ray chest was done to rule out pneumothorax. Patient (or responsible adult) was given post-procedure and discharge instructions to follow at home. The patient was discharged in stable condition after making a follow-up appointment.

Pre-procedure pain score: _____

Post-procedure pain score: _____

CHAPTER 2

ACROMIOCLAVICULAR JOINT INJECTION

Name: _____ age/sex _____ date/time _____

PROCEDURE: Acromioclavicular joint injection under Fluoroscopic guidance, left/right side

DIAGNOSIS: _____

PHYSICIAN: _____

MEDICATIONS INJECTED: 0.5 ml of Triamcinolone/Methylprednisolone (20 mg) and 0.5 ml of 1% Lignocaine/0.25% Bupivacaine

SEDATION MEDICATIONS: None

ANAESTHESIA: Local/sedation/TIVA/General Anesthesia

COMPLICATIONS: None

TECHNIQUE: After confirming written informed consent and NPO status, multipara monitor was attached to the patient. Time-out was taken to identify the correct patient, procedure and side prior to starting the procedure.

With the patient lying in the supine position, the parts were prepped and draped in the usual sterile fashion using betadine-spirit and sterile fenestrated drape. Medial edge of the acromion, lateral edge of the clavicle and acromioclavicular joint was identified on fluoroscopy in AP view.

A 25-gauge, 2-inch needle was inserted at the AC joint. It was then advanced parallel to the floor towards the acromioclavicular joint using intermittent fluoroscopy. Once the tip reached the intraarticular space, 0.5 ml Omnipaque 240 was injected after negative aspiration for blood. Intraarticular spread was confirmed with no vascular uptake. At this point, treatment medication was injected slowly. Needle was removed intact. A sterile dressing was applied.

The procedure was completed without complications and was tolerated well. After the procedure, the patient was monitored for 30 minutes in the recovery room. The patient (or responsible adult) was given post-procedure and discharge instructions to follow at home. The patient was discharged in stable condition after making a follow-up appointment.

Pre-procedure pain score: _____

Post-procedure pain score: _____

CHAPTER 3

GLENOHUMERAL JOINT INJECTION
ANTERIOR APPROACH

Name: _____ age/sex _____ date/time _____

PROCEDURE: Glenohumeral joint injection anterior approach under fluoroscopy guidance, left/right side

DIAGNOSIS: _____

PHYSICIAN: _____

MEDICATIONS INJECTED: 4 ml of 0.125% Bupivacaine with 1 ml (40 mg) Methylprednisolone/Triamcinolone

ANAESTHESIA: Local/sedation/TIVA/General Anesthesia

SEDATION MEDICATIONS: None

COMPLICATIONS: None

TECHNIQUE: After confirming written informed consent, multipara monitor was attached to the patient. Time-out was taken to identify the correct patient, procedure and side prior to starting the procedure.

Patient was positioned supine with arm supinated and kept by the side of body. Parts were prepped and draped in the usual sterile fashion using betadine-spirit and sterile fenestrated drape. Glenohumeral joint was kept in center of image intensifier in AP view. Entry point was marked at the anteromedial part of humeral head in line with coracoid process (at 10-12'O clock for left shoulder and 12-2'O clock for right shoulder). 3 ml of 2% Lignocaine was infiltrated in skin, subcutaneous tissue using 25-gauge needle.

A 25-gauge 2-inch needle was inserted at the entry point with bevel facing inwards and advanced vertically in tunnel view under intermittent fluoroscopy till it hit humeral head. A give way was felt as needle crossed the joint capsule. Needle position was confirmed to be at the edge of humeral head near top of Glenohumeral joint in AP view. Aspiration was attempted to rule out intravascular placement. 1 ml of Omnipaque 240 was then injected. Contrast was seen along the joint line, following contour of humeral head, it spread subcapsular and to inferior recess thus confirming intraarticular position of the needle. There was no vascular runoff. Medication was then injected slowly.

The procedure was completed without complications and was tolerated well. After the procedure, the patient was monitored for 30 minutes in the recovery room. The patient (or responsible adult) was given post-procedure and discharge instructions to follow at home. The patient was discharged in stable condition after making a follow-up appointment.

Pre-procedure pain score: _____

Post-procedure pain score: _____

CHAPTER 4

GLENOHUMERAL JOINT INJECTION
POSTERIOR APPROACH

Name: _____ age/sex _____date/time _____

PROCEDURE: Glenohumeral joint injection posterior approach, landmark guided, left/right side

DIAGNOSIS: _____

PHYSICIAN: _____

MEDICATIONS INJECTED: 4 ml of 0.125% Bupivacaine/ 1%Lignocaine with 40 mg Methylprednisolone/Triamcinolone

ANAESTHESIA: Local/sedation/TIVA/General Anesthesia

SEDATION MEDICATIONS: None

COMPLICATIONS: None

TECHNIQUE: After confirming written informed consent, multipara monitor was attached to the patient. Time-out was taken to identify the correct patient, procedure and side prior to starting the procedure.

Patient was positioned sitting at the edge of bed with arm hanging off. Parts were prepped and draped in the usual sterile fashion using betadine-spirit and sterile fenestrated drape. Posterior corner of acromion and coracoid process was palpated. Entry point was marked 2 fingerbreadths inferior and 2 fingerbreadths medial to posterior corner of acromion. 2% Lignocaine was infiltrated in skin, subcutaneous tissue using 25-gauge needle.

A 22-gauge 1.5-inch needle was inserted at the entry point with bevel facing upwards and advanced anteriorly, medially aiming for coracoid process. A give way was felt as needle crossed the joint capsule. Aspiration was attempted to confirm intraarticular placement and to rule out vascular placement. Medication was then injected slowly; it could be injected freely.

The procedure was completed without complications and was tolerated well. After the procedure, the patient was monitored for 30 minutes in the recovery room. The patient (or responsible adult) was given post-procedure and discharge instructions to follow at home. The patient was discharged in stable condition after making a follow-up appointment.

Pre-procedure pain score: _____

Post-procedure pain score: _____

CHAPTER 5

SUBACROMIAL INJECTION

Name: _____ age/sex _____ date/time _____

PROCEDURE: Subacromial injections, landmark guided, left/right side

DIAGNOSIS: _____

PHYSICIAN: _____

MEDICATIONS INJECTED: 4 ml of 0.125% Bupivacaine with 40 mg Methylprednisolone/Triamcinolone

ANAESTHESIA: Local/sedation/TIVA/General Anesthesia

SEDATION MEDICATIONS: None

COMPLICATIONS: None

TECHNIQUE: After confirming written informed consent, multipara monitor was attached to the patient. Time-out was taken to identify the correct patient, procedure and side prior to starting the procedure.

Patient was positioned sitting at the edge of bed with arm hanging off. Parts were prepped and draped in the usual sterile fashion using betadine-spirit and sterile fenestrated drape. Posterior corner of acromion process was palpated. Entry point was 1 cm below the edge of posterior border of acromion, just medial to posterior corner of acromion. 2% Lignocaine was infiltrated in skin, subcutaneous tissue up-to joint capsule using 25-gauge needle.

A 22-gauge 1.5-inch needle was inserted at the entry point with bevel facing upwards and advanced anteriorly, medially and slightly superiorly aiming for midpoint of acromion process. Aspiration was attempted to confirm intraarticular placement and to rule out vascular placement. Medication was then injected slowly; it could be injected freely.

The procedure was completed without complications and was tolerated well. After the procedure, the patient was monitored for 30 minutes in the recovery room. The patient (or responsible adult) was given post-procedure and discharge instructions to follow at home. The patient was discharged in stable condition after making a follow-up appointment.

Pre-procedure pain score: _____

Post-procedure pain score: _____

CHAPTER 6

INTERCOSTAL NERVE BLOCK

Name: _____ age/sex _____ date/time _____

PROCEDURE: Fluoroscopy guided Intercostal nerve block, ...levels, left/right side

DIAGNOSIS: _____

PHYSICIAN: _____

MEDICATIONS INJECTED: 1 ml (40 mg) Methylprednisolone/Triamcinolone with 9 ml of 1% Lignocaine, 3 ml at each level

SEDATION MEDICATIONS: none

ANAESTHESIA: Local/sedation/TIVA/General Anesthesia

COMPLICATIONS: None

TECHNIQUE: After confirming written informed consent and NPO status, multipara monitor was attached to the patient. Intravenous access was secured. Time-out was taken to identify the correct patient, procedure and side prior to starting the procedure.

Patient was placed prone. Parts were prepped and draped in the usual sterile fashion using betadine-spirit and sterile fenestrated drape.

Rib at the level of targeted intercostal nerve was fluoroscopically visualized in AP view. Angle of rib is marked. A 25-gauge, 2-inch needle was used to proceed down to the inferior aspect of the rib lateral to the angle. The needle was then walked off inferiorly until it dipped down to just below the rib. After a negative aspiration, Omnipaque 240 contrast was used to confirm spread along the under surface of the desired rib. Treatment medication was then given at this level. Similar procedure was repeated at other levels. Needle was removed intact. Sterile dressing was applied.

The procedure was completed without complications and was tolerated well. After the procedure, the patient was monitored for 2 hours in the recovery room. An X-ray chest was done before discharge. The patient (or responsible adult) was given post-procedure and discharge instructions to follow at home. The patient was discharged in stable condition after making a follow-up appointment.

Pre-procedure pain score: _____

Post-procedure pain score: _____

SECTION 7
HEAD, FACE AND NECK

CHAPTER 1

STELLATE GANGLION BLOCK AT C6

Name: _____ age/sex _____ date/time _____

PROCEDURE: Stellate Ganglion block under Fluoroscopic guidance, left/right side

DIAGNOSIS: _____

PHYSICIAN: _____

MEDICATIONS INJECTED: 10 ml 0.25% Bupivacaine

ANAESTHESIA: Local anesthesia/local anesthesia with sedation/TIVA/General anesthesia

SEDATION MEDICATIONS: None

COMPLICATIONS: None

TECHNIQUE: After confirming written informed consent and NPO status, multipara monitor was attached to the patient. Surface thermometry probe was attached on both the upper extremities. Intravenous access was secured. Time-out was taken to identify the correct patient, procedure and side prior to starting the procedure.

Patient was positioned supine with a shoulder roll for extension of neck. Parts were prepped and draped in the usual sterile fashion using betadine-spirit and sterile fenestrated drape.

Chassaignac's tubercle and the transverse process of the 6th cervical vertebra was identified in AP view of fluoroscopy. Sternocleidomastoid and carotid sheath was displaced laterally. Once the carotid sheath was out of the way, a 22-gauge needle was inserted perpendicularly to all planes and advanced till bony contact was made with of Chassaignac's tubercle on the transverse process of 6th cervical vertebra. Needle was then withdrawn 1-2 mm and held steady with left hand. After negative aspiration for blood and CSF, 2 ml of Omnipaque 240 was injected. It was seen at the lateral borders of the ipsilateral cervical vertebral bodies on AP view. Treatment medication was then injected in aliquots of 2 cc with negative aspirations between injections. Needle was removed intact. Pressure was placed over the puncture site for approximately five minutes. A sterile dressing was applied.

The procedure was completed without complications and was tolerated well. Patient was given head-up position for 15 minutes. Patient had Horner's sign after the block was established. After the procedure, the patient was monitored for 2 hours in the recovery room. Monitoring was done for hemodynamic stability, Skin temperature, Sensory/ motor function of upper extremity, Vasodilation, change of color, decreased sweating, and pain reduction. Patient was kept NPO for 4 hours post-procedure. The patient (or responsible adult) was given post-procedure and discharge instructions to follow at home. The patient was discharged in stable condition after making a follow-up appointment

Right upper extremity: Pre-injection skin temp = _____ Post-injection skin temp=_____

Left upper extremity: Pre-injection skin temp= _____ Post-injection skin temp= _____

Pre-procedure pain score: _____

Post-procedure pain score: _____

CHAPTER 2

STELLATE GANGLION BLOCK AT C7

Name: _____ age/sex _____ date/time _____

PROCEDURE: Stellate Ganglion block under Fluoroscopic guidance, left/right side

DIAGNOSIS: _____

PHYSICIAN: _____

MEDICATIONS INJECTED: Bupivacaine 0.25%- 2 ml for sympathetic block of head, face and neck or 5 ml for T2-T3 block

ANAESTHESIA: Local anesthesia/ local anesthesia with sedation/ TIVA/ General anesthesia

SEDATION MEDICATIONS: None

COMPLICATIONS: None

TECHNIQUE: After confirming written informed consent and NPO status, multipara monitor was attached to the patient. Surface thermometry probe was attached on both the upper extremities. Intravenous access was secured. Time-out was taken to identify the correct patient, procedure and side prior to starting the procedure.

Patient was positioned supine with a shoulder roll for extension of neck. Parts were prepped and draped in the usual sterile fashion using betadine-spirit and sterile fenestrated drape.

C7 vertebral body was visualized in AP view. Image intensifier was rotated ipsilateral oblique to visualize uncinate process of C7. The carotid sheath was retracted laterally with non-dominant hand. 22-gauge needle was inserted at the junction of uncinate process with the C7 vertebral body and advanced end-on till it made bony contact. Needle position was confirmed to be at the base of uncinate process in AP and oblique view. Dye spread at the anterolateral border of vertebral body was confirmed on AP view after injecting 2 ml of Omnipaque 240. Then treatment medication was injected after negative aspiration for blood and CSF. Needle was removed intact. Pressure was placed over the puncture site for approximately five minutes. A sterile dressing was applied.

The procedure was completed without complications and was tolerated well. Patient was given head-up position for 15 minutes. Patient had Horner's sign after the block was established. After the procedure, the patient was monitored for 2 hours in the recovery room. Monitoring was done for hemodynamic stability, Skin temperature, Sensory/ motor function of upper extremity, Vasodilation, change of color, decreased sweating, and pain reduction. Patient was kept NPO for 4 hours post-procedure. The patient (or responsible adult) was given post-procedure and discharge instructions to follow at home. The patient was discharged in stable condition after making a follow-up appointment

Right upper extremity: Pre-injection skin temp = _____ Post-injection skin temp=_____

Left upper extremity: Pre-injection skin temp= _____ Post-injection skin temp= _____

Pre-procedure pain score: _____

Post-procedure pain score: _____

CHAPTER 3

MAXILLARY NERVE BLOCK

Name: _____ age/sex _____ date/time _____

PROCEDURE: Maxillary nerve block under Fluoroscopic guidance, left/right side

DIAGNOSIS: _____

PHYSICIAN: _____

MEDICATIONS INJECTED: 5 ml of 1% Lignocaine/0.25% Bupivacaine

SEDATION MEDICATIONS: None

ANAESTHESIA: Local/sedation/TIVA/General Anesthesia

COMPLICATIONS: None

TECHNIQUE: After confirming written informed consent, multipara monitor was attached to the patient. Time-out was taken to identify the correct patient, procedure and side prior to starting the procedure.

Patient was positioned supine with the head in a neutral position. Parts were prepped and draped in the usual sterile fashion using betadine-spirit and sterile fenestrated drape.

The patient was asked to open and close his mouth few times to facilitate palpation of the Coronoid notch just anterior and below the tragus of the ear. On fluoroscopy in lateral view, coronoid notch was identified between the coronoid and condylar processes of the ramus of the mandible below zygomatic arch. Needle entry point was marked as high as possible in the space between the zygomatic arch and the center of the coronoid notch. 2% Lignocaine was infiltrated in skin, subcutaneous tissue using 25-gauge needle.

A 23-gauge spinal needle was introduced under fluoroscopic guidance at the site already marked and advanced in a horizontal plane perpendicular to skin. Needle was advanced till it touched lateral pterygoid plate. Depth was noted (4-5 cm) and needle was withdrawn by 2-3mm. Then the needle was redirected slightly superior and anterior up to the same noted depth, to walk off the lateral pterygoid plate. Paresthesia was elicited in the maxillary nerve distribution (nose ridge, upper lip, gum, and face). After negative aspiration of blood and CSF, 1 ml Omnipaque 240 was injected to confirm the position of needle. Then treatment medication was injected slowly. Needle was removed intact. Sterile dressing was applied.

The procedure was completed without complications and was tolerated well. After the procedure, the patient was monitored for 2 hours in the recovery room. The patient (or responsible adult) was given post-procedure and discharge instructions to follow at home. The patient was discharged in stable condition after making a follow-up appointment.

Pre-procedure pain score: _____

Post-procedure pain score: _____

CHAPTER 4

MANDIBULAR NERVE BLOCK

Name: _____ age/sex _____ date/time _____

PROCEDURE: Mandibular nerve block under Fluoroscopic guidance, left/right side

DIAGNOSIS: _____

PHYSICIAN: _____

MEDICATIONS INJECTED: 3 ml of 1% Lignocaine/0.25% Bupivacaine

SEDATION MEDICATIONS: None

ANAESTHESIA: Local/sedation/TIVA/General Anesthesia

COMPLICATIONS: None

TECHNIQUE: After confirming written informed consent, multipara monitor was attached to the patient. Time-out was taken to identify the correct patient, procedure and side prior to starting the procedure.

Patient was positioned supine with the head in a neutral position. Parts were prepped and draped in the usual sterile fashion using betadine-spirit and sterile fenestrated drape. The patient was asked to open and close his mouth few times to facilitate palpation of the Coronoid notch just anterior and below the tragus of the ear. Coronoid notch was located between the coronoid and condylar processes of the ramus of the mandible below zygomatic arch in lateral view on fluoroscopy. Needle entry point was marked as high as possible in the space between the zygomatic arch and the center of the coronoid notch. 2% Lignocaine was infiltrated in skin, subcutaneous tissue using 25-gauge needle.

A 23-gauge spinal needle was introduced under fluoroscopic guidance at the site already marked and advanced in a horizontal plane perpendicular to skin. Needle was advanced till it touched lateral pterygoid plate. Depth was noted (4-5 cm) and needle was withdrawn by 2-3mm. Then the needle was redirected slightly inferior and posterior up to the same noted depth, to walk off the lateral pterygoid plate. Paresthesia was elicited in the mandibular nerve distribution (lower mandible, lower lip, lower jaw, and tongue). After negative aspiration of blood and CSF, 1 ml Omnipaque 240 was injected to confirm the position of needle. Then treatment medication was injected slowly. Needle was removed intact. Sterile dressing was applied.

The procedure was completed without complications and was tolerated well. After the procedure, the patient was monitored for 2 hours in the recovery room. The patient (or responsible adult) was given post-procedure and discharge instructions to follow at home. The patient was discharged in stable condition after making a follow-up appointment.

Pre-procedure pain score: _____

Post-procedure pain score: _____

CHAPTER 5

SUPRAORBITAL AND SUPRATROCHLEAR NERVE BLOCK

Name: _____ age/sex _____date/time _____

PROCEDURE: **Landmark Technique for supraorbital and supratrochlear nerve block,** left/right side

DIAGNOSIS: _____

PHYSICIAN: _____

MEDICATIONS INJECTED: 0.5 ml of 1% Lignocaine/0.25% Bupivacaine at each site

SEDATION MEDICATIONS: None

ANAESTHESIA: Local/sedation/TIVA/General Anesthesia

COMPLICATIONS: None

TECHNIQUE: After confirming written informed consent, multipara monitor was attached to the patient. Time-out was taken to identify the correct patient, procedure and side prior to starting the procedure.

Patient was positioned supine with the head in a neutral position. Parts were prepped and draped in the usual sterile fashion using betadine-spirit and sterile fenestrated drape.

Supraorbital foramen was palpated by following the orbit rim 2 cm from the midline, at the intersection of the medial one-third and the lateral two-thirds. A 25-gauge intradermal needle was introduced 0.5 cm under the inferior edge of the eyebrow, perpendicular to the skin, and was directed medially and cephalad. When the needle tip was near the supraorbital notch, after test aspiration, and with caution not to penetrate the foramen, treatment medication was injected, creating a subcutaneous wheal.

The supratrochlear nerve was blocked immediately following supraorbital nerve block, without removing the needle, by directing the needle about 1 cm toward the midline. The landmark was marked at the top of the angle formed by the eyebrow and the nasal spine. An additional 0.5 ml of treatment medication was injected. Needle was removed intact. Firm pressure was applied for 5 minutes and then sterile dressing was applied.

The procedure was completed without complications and was tolerated well. After the procedure, the patient was monitored for 30 minutes in the recovery room. The patient (or responsible adult) was given post-procedure and discharge instructions to follow at home. The patient was discharged in stable condition after making a follow-up appointment.

Pre-procedure pain score: _____

Post-procedure pain score: _____

CHAPTER 6

MAXILLARY NERVE RADIOFREQUENCY ABLATION

Name: _____ age/sex _____ date/time _____

PROCEDURE: Maxillary nerve radiofrequency ablation under Fluoroscopic guidance, left/right side

DIAGNOSIS: _____

PHYSICIAN: _____

MEDICATIONS INJECTED: 2 ml of 2% Lignocaine/0. 5% Bupivacaine

SEDATION MEDICATIONS: None

ANAESTHESIA: Local/sedation/TIVA/General Anesthesia

COMPLICATIONS: None

TECHNIQUE: After confirming written informed consent, multipara monitor was attached to the patient. Time-out was taken to identify the correct patient, procedure and side prior to starting the procedure.

Patient was positioned supine with the head in a neutral position. Parts were prepped and draped in the usual sterile fashion using betadine-spirit and sterile fenestrated drape. The patient was asked to open and close his mouth few times to facilitate palpation of the Coronoid notch just anterior and below the tragus of the ear. Coronoid notch was located between the coronoid and condylar processes of the ramus of the mandible below zygomatic arch on fluoroscopy in lateral view. Needle entry point was marked as high as possible in the space between the zygomatic arch and the center of the coronoid notch. 2% Lignocaine was infiltrated in skin, subcutaneous tissue using 25-gauge needle.

A 22-gauge radiofrequency needle, 10 cm long, with 5 mm active tip was introduced under fluoroscopic guidance at the site already marked and advanced in a horizontal plane perpendicular to skin. Needle was advanced till it touched lateral pterygoid plate. Depth was noted (4-5 cm) and needle was withdrawn by 2-3mm. Then the needle was redirected slightly superior and anterior up to the same noted depth, to walk off the lateral pterygoid plate. 1 ml Omnipaque 240 was injected to confirm the position of needle. Sensory stimulation of 50Hz at 0.5 V elicited paresthesia in the maxillary distribution (nose ridge, upper lip, gum, and face). There was no motor stimulation at 2Hz. After negative aspiration of blood and CSF, 2 ml of 2% Lignocaine/ 0.5% Bupivacaine was injected slowly. Lesioning was done at 80⁰C for 90 sec. Needle was removed intact. Sterile dressing was applied.

The procedure was completed without complications and was tolerated well. Patient was assessed for weakness and numbness of jaw. After the procedure, the patient was monitored for 2 hours in the recovery room. The patient (or responsible adult) was given post-procedure and discharge instructions to follow at home. The patient was discharged in stable condition after making a follow-up appointment.

Pre-procedure pain score: _____

Post-procedure pain score: _____

CHAPTER 7

MANDIBULAR NERVE RADIOFREQUENCY ABLATION

Name: _____ age/sex _____date/time _____

PROCEDURE: Mandibular nerve radiofrequency ablation under Fluoroscopic guidance, left/right side

DIAGNOSIS: _____

PHYSICIAN: _____

MEDICATIONS INJECTED: 2 ml of 2% Lignocaine/0. 5% Bupivacaine

SEDATION MEDICATIONS: None

ANAESTHESIA: Local/sedation/TIVA/General Anesthesia

COMPLICATIONS: None

TECHNIQUE: After confirming written informed consent, multipara monitor was attached to the patient. Time-out was taken to identify the correct patient, procedure and side prior to starting the procedure.

Patient was positioned supine with the head in a neutral position. Parts were prepped and draped in the usual sterile fashion using betadine-spirit and sterile fenestrated drape. The patient was asked to open and close his mouth few times to facilitate palpation of the Coronoid notch just anterior and below the tragus of the ear. Coronoid notch was located between the coronoid and condylar processes of the ramus of the mandible below zygomatic arch on fluoroscopy in lateral view. Needle entry point was marked as high as possible in the space between the zygomatic arch and the center of the coronoid notch. 2% Lignocaine was infiltrated in skin, subcutaneous tissue using 25-gauge needle.

A 22-gauge radiofrequency needle, 10 cm long, with 5 mm active tip was introduced under fluoroscopic guidance at the site already marked and advanced in a horizontal plane perpendicular to skin. Needle was advanced till it touched lateral pterygoid plate. Depth was noted (4-5 cm) and needle was withdrawn by 2-3mm. Then the needle was redirected slightly inferior and posterior up to the same noted depth, to walk off the lateral pterygoid plate. 1 ml Omnipaque 240 was injected to confirm the position of needle. Sensory stimulation of 50Hz at 0.5 V elicited paresthesia in the mandibular distribution (lower mandible, lower lip, lower jaw, and tongue). After negative aspiration of blood and CSF, 2 ml of 2% Lignocaine/ 0.5% Bupivacaine was injected slowly. Lesioning was done at 80°C for 90 sec. Needle was removed intact. Sterile dressing was applied.

The procedure was completed without complications and was tolerated well. Patient was assessed for weakness and numbness of jaw. After the procedure, the patient was monitored for 2 hours in the recovery room. The patient (or responsible adult) was given post-procedure and discharge instructions to follow at home. The patient was discharged in stable condition after making a follow-up appointment.

Pre-procedure pain score: _____

Post-procedure pain score: _____

CHAPTER 8

GASSERIAN GANGLION BLOCK

Name: _____ age/sex _____date/time _____

PROCEDURE: Fluoroscopy guided Gasserian ganglion block, left/right side

DIAGNOSIS: _____

PHYSICIAN: _____

MEDICATIONS INJECTED:

SEDATION MEDICATIONS: 1.5 mg Midazolam, 100mcg Fentanyl, 5+2+2+2 ml Propofol

ANAESTHESIA: Local/sedation/TIVA/General Anesthesia

COMPLICATIONS: None

TECHNIQUE: After confirming written informed consent and NPO status, multipara monitor was attached to the patient. Intravenous access was secured. Time-out was taken to identify the correct patient, procedure and side prior to starting the procedure.

Patient was placed supine with neck extended, chin up-looking at ceiling. Parts were prepped and draped in the usual sterile fashion using betadine-spirit and sterile fenestrated drape. Initially AP view was obtained then image intensifier was tilted caudal and ipsilateral oblique to get a Submental view. Rising sun sign was seen by decreasing caudal tilt in real-time fluoroscopy. Foramen Ovale is identified as an oval structure, lateral to maxillary sinus, medial to mandibular condyle. Entry site was marked at the foramen ovale, 2 cm lateral to angle of mouth for V2-V3, and 3 cm lateral to angle of mouth for V1. Local anesthetic 5 ml of 1% Lignocaine was given at the entry site by raising a skin wheal and along path of RF needle using a 26-gauge 1.25-inch needle.

22-gauge, 10 cm, RF needle with 5 mm active tip, tip bent was inserted at the entry point with curve lateral to avoid piercing cheek. Needle was advanced in tunnel view on foramen ovale, Needle was directed towards middle of pupil. Needle was aimed towards middle third of foramen for V2/V3, and medial third of foramen for V1. Needle was advanced till it hit the bone (lateral margin of ovale). then needle tip was turned medially to enter the foramen ovale. When at ovale, patient complained of pain in V3 distribution. Needle depth was checked in lateral view. Needle was advanced slowly under intermittent fluoroscopy in lateral view till it reached junction of horizontal portion of petrous and clival line. Needle tip was 2 mm above the line for V1, at the line for V2, and 2mm below the line for V3.

Using Radiofrequency machine, Impedance was 200-800. Motor stimulation at 2 Hz showed no movement. With sensory stimulation at 50Hz patient experienced paresthesia of the affected division at 0.05-0.2 V. First lesioning was done at 60^0 for 60 sec. Second lesioning was done at 65^0 for 60 sec and then at 70^0 for 60 sec. Sensory stimulation was checked before each lesioning.

Needle was removed intact and pressure was applied at the needle insertion site for 2 minutes. Patient was asked to apply ice pack afterwards.

After the procedure, the patient was monitored in the recovery room. Patient was assessed for cheek hematoma. Sensory (numbness), motor (jaw closure) and corneal reflex after V1 assessment was done. The procedure was completed without complications and was tolerated well. The patient (or responsible adult) was given discharge instructions to follow at home. The patient was discharged next day in stable condition after making a follow-up appointment.

Pre-procedure pain score: _____

Post-procedure pain score: _____

CHAPTER 9

SPHENOPALATINE GANGLION BLOCK

Name: _____ age/sex _____ date/time _____

PROCEDURE: Sphenopalatine ganglion block under Fluoroscopic guidance, left/right side

DIAGNOSIS: _____

PHYSICIAN: _____

MEDICATIONS INJECTED: 1 ml of 2% Lignocaine/0. 5% Bupivacaine

SEDATION MEDICATIONS: None

ANAESTHESIA: Local/sedation/TIVA/General Anesthesia

COMPLICATIONS: None

TECHNIQUE: After confirming written informed consent, multipara monitor was attached to the patient. Time-out was taken to identify the correct patient, procedure and side prior to starting the procedure.

Patient was positioned supine with the head in a neutral position. Parts were prepped and draped in the usual sterile fashion using betadine-spirit and sterile fenestrated drape.

Temporomandibular joint and external auditory meatus was visualized in lateral view on fluoroscopy. Image intensifier was rotated to overlap temporomandibular joint and external auditory meatus of both the sides. Pterygopalatine fossa was seen as inverted vas posterior to maxillary sinus and just anterior to end of petrous part of temporal bone. Coronoid notch was located between the coronoid and condylar processes of the ramus of the mandible below zygomatic arch on fluoroscopy in lateral view. Needle entry point was marked as high as possible in the space between the zygomatic arch and the center of the coronoid notch. 2% Lignocaine was infiltrated in skin, subcutaneous tissue using 25-gauge needle.

A 22-gauge radiofrequency needle, 10 cm long, with 5 mm active tip was introduced under fluoroscopic guidance at the entry point and advanced in a superior, medial and anterior direction towards the inverted vas. Depth of needle was confirmed on AP view, needle was not crossing the lateral nasal border and was at the supero-medial end of maxillary sinus. After negative aspiration of blood and CSF, 1 ml of 2% Lignocaine/ 0.5% Bupivacaine was injected slowly. Sensory stimulation was done at 50 Hz at 0.6V, patient felt it in the nose and base of nose. Lesioning was done at...80°C for 90 sec.............Needle was removed intact. Sterile dressing was applied.

The procedure was completed without complications and was tolerated well. After the procedure, the patient was monitored for 2 hours in the recovery room. The patient (or responsible adult) was given post-procedure and discharge instructions to follow at home. The patient was discharged in stable condition after making a follow-up appointment.

Pre-procedure pain score: _____

Post-procedure pain score: _____

CHAPTER 10

GLOSSOPHARYNGEAL NERVE BLOCK

Name: _____ age/sex _____date/time _____

PROCEDURE: Glossopharyngeal nerve block under Fluoroscopic guidance, left/right side

DIAGNOSIS: _____

PHYSICIAN: _____

MEDICATIONS INJECTED: 3 ml of 2% Lignocaine

SEDATION MEDICATIONS: None

ANAESTHESIA: Local/sedation/TIVA/General Anesthesia

COMPLICATIONS: None

TECHNIQUE: After confirming written informed consent, multipara monitor was attached to the patient. Time-out was taken to identify the correct patient, procedure and side prior to starting the procedure.

Patient was positioned supine with the head slightly rotated to opposite side. Parts were prepped and draped in the usual sterile fashion using betadine-spirit and sterile fenestrated drape. Styloid process was identified midway between mastoid process and angle of mandible in lateral view on fluoroscopy.

22-gauge blunt tip needle advanced perpendicular to skin towards the posterior aspect of styloid process. After hitting the bone at ....cm, needle was withdrawn by 2 mm and was walked off posteriorly. After aspirating to rule out blood or CSF, 1 ml Omnipaque 240 was injected in real time fluoroscopy to rule out vascular run off. 3 ml of 2% Lignocaine was injected in 1 ml increments. Needle was removed intact. Sterile dressing was applied.

The procedure was completed without complications and was tolerated well. After the procedure, the patient was monitored for 4 hours in the recovery room. Patient was assessed for hoarseness, trapezius weakness and tongue weakness (cranial nerves X, XI, XII). Patient was kept NBM for 4 hours after the procedure. The patient (or responsible adult) was given post-procedure and discharge instructions to follow at home. The patient was discharged in stable condition after making a follow-up appointment.

Pre-procedure pain score: _____

Post-procedure pain score: _____

SECTION 8
ALTERNATE THERAPIES

CHAPTER 1

MYOFASCIAL TRIGGER POINT INJECTION

Name: _____ age/sex _____date/time _____

PROCEDURE: Myofascial Trigger Point injection (MTrP), _____
muscle, left/right side

DIAGNOSIS: _____

PHYSICIAN: _____

MEDICATIONS INJECTED: Total ....ml of 1%Lignocaine/ 0.25% Bupivacaine with 40
mg Triamcinolone/Methylprednisolone

SEDATION MEDICATIONS: None

ANAESTHESIA: None/ local

COMPLICATIONS: None

TECHNIQUE: After confirming written informed consent, multipara monitor was attached to the patient. Time-out was taken to identify the correct patient, procedure and side prior to starting the procedure.

Patient was positioned prone/ Supine/ right lateral/ left lateral. Patient was asked to remain immobile during the procedure. Parts were prepped and draped in the usual sterile fashion using betadine-spirit and sterile fenestrated drape.

Taut band of muscle was palpated. Myofascial Trigger point (MTrP) was palpated as the most tender region in the taut band of muscle. Vapocoolant spray was sprayed for 5 seconds from a distance of about 45 cm to provide cold anesthesia and was allowed to evaporate from skin.

Skin was pulled taut to hold MTrP in position. 22-gauge, 1.5-inch needle attached to the syringe containing treatment medication was then introduced through the skin into the trigger point. Needle was inserted quickly to fully penetrate the taut band, medication was injected and then pulled back up to subcutaneous tissue and reinserted again in other direction. Fast-in, fast out technique was used. Total ....ml of 1%Lignocaine/ 0.25% Bupivacaine with 40 mg Triamcinolone/Methylprednisolone was injected. After inactivating all the trigger points, needle was removed intact and pressure was applied for 5 minutes. A full active stretch of the _____ muscle was performed.

The procedure was completed without complications and was tolerated well. After the procedure, the patient was monitored for 30 minutes in the recovery room. The patient (or responsible adult) was given post-procedure and discharge instructions to follow at home. The patient was discharged in stable condition after making a follow-up appointment.

Pre-procedure pain score: _____

Post-procedure pain score: _____

CHAPTER 2

INTRAMUSCULAR STIMULATION

Name: _____ age/sex _____ date/time _____

PROCEDURE: Intramuscular Stimulation of _____ muscle, left/right side

DIAGNOSIS: _____

PHYSICIAN: _____

MEDICATIONS INJECTED: None

SEDATION MEDICATIONS: None

ANAESTHESIA: None

COMPLICATIONS: None

TECHNIQUE: After confirming written informed consent, multipara monitor was attached to the patient. Time-out was taken to identify the correct patient, procedure and side prior to starting the procedure.

Patient was positioned prone/ supine/ right lateral/ left lateral. Patient was asked to remain immobile during the procedure. Parts were prepped and draped in the usual sterile fashion using betadine-spirit and sterile fenestrated drape.

Taut band of muscle was palpated. Myofascial Trigger point was palpated as the most tender region in the taut band of muscle. Taut band was fixed with fingers. Filiform solid IMS needle (.............mm) in the plastic sheath was held in non-dominant hand and a gentle tap was given at the needle hub by dominant hand so that the needle pierced the skin. The needle was then guided deeper by a gentle twirling motion. Loss of resistance was felt indicating needle entry into the taut muscle. Local twitch response was seen. Jump sign positive. In total, ... needles were inserted in the......................................muscle. Needles were grasped tightly in the muscle.

Needles were removed after 20 minutes. Needles could be removed easily indicating relaxation of the muscle. All the needles were removed intact.

The procedure was completed without complications and was tolerated well. After the procedure, the patient was monitored for 30 minutes in the recovery room. The patient (or responsible adult) was given post-procedure and discharge instructions to follow at home. The patient was discharged in stable condition after making a follow-up appointment.

Pre-procedure pain score: _____

Post-procedure pain score: _____

SECTION 9
ANNEXURE

CHAPTER 1

INFORMED CONSENT FORM

Name: _____ age/sex _____ date/time _____

PROCEDURE: _____

DIAGNOSIS: _____

PHYSICIAN: _____

The intended <u>benefits</u> of the procedure: Relief of symptoms/ identify source of pain/

_____

Serious or frequently occurring <u>risks</u> include Bleeding, infection, bruising/tenderness, pain flair, temporary numbness and/or weakness, pain at injection site, allergic reaction

_____

If you decide not to have this procedure, your <u>alternative</u> option is to continue to manage the pain conservatively using medicines and physiotherapy _____

Potential <u>risks of not receiving treatment</u>: _____

Relative <u>chances of success</u> of procedure: _____

I have been explained about the procedure, possible benefits, risks and alternatives available to me, chances of success of the procedure in the language I understand. I hereby authorize and give my voluntary consent to the physician _____ for performing the intervention _____ for treatment of my pain.

Patient's name: _____

Sign _____

Date _____

Witness name: _____

Sign _____

Date _____

CHAPTER 2

RESUSCITATION CART CONTENTS

Always keep following equipments and drugs readily available in the procedure room

- Oxygen (preferably pipeline/ an "E"-size cylinder)

- Suction, suction catheter

- AMBU bag

- Airway management devices: masks, Laryngoscope, Endotracheal tubes, oropharyngeal airways, LMAs

- Drugs: Adrenaline, Atropine, Amiodarone, Chlorpheniramine, Diphenhydramine, Dopamine, Noradrenaline, Nitroglycerine, Aspirin, Sorbitrate, Hydrocortisone, Salbutamol inhaler and respules, Oral carbohydrate source, Ephedrine, preservative free Lignocaine, 25% Dextrose, Magnesium sulphate, Sodium bicarbonate, Calcium chloride, Propofol, Glucagon

- Lipid emulsion 20%

- Nebulizer

- IV fluids

- Defibrillator/ AED

CHAPTER 3

ASRA GUIDELINES FOR LOCAL ANESTHETIC SYSTEMIC TOXICITY

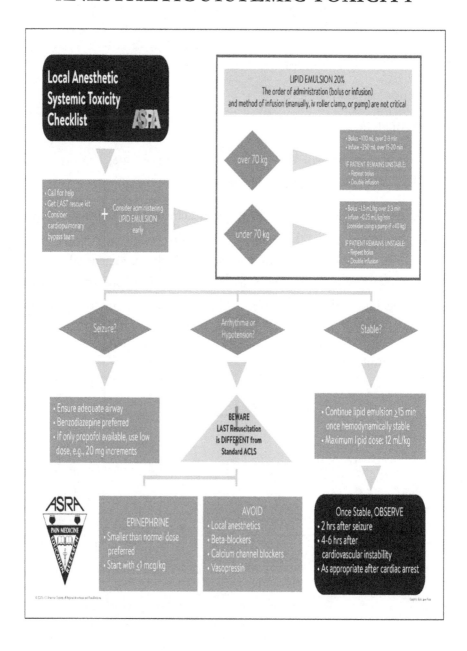

CHAPTER 4

EMERGENCY MANAGEMENT OF ANAPHYLAXIS

- Remove allergen (if still present).

- Call for assistance.

- **Lay patient flat.** Do not allow them to stand or walk. If breathing is difficult, allow them to sit.

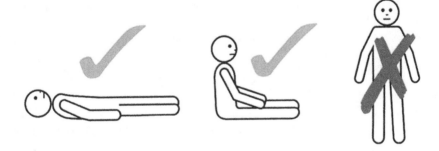

- **Give** intramuscular **injection (IMI)** adrenaline (1:1000) **into outer mid-thigh** (0.01mg/kg = 0.5mg per dose) without delay

- If multiple doses are required for a severe reaction (e.g., 2-3 doses administered at 5-minute intervals), consider adrenaline infusion if skills and equipment are available.

- Give oxygen.

- Call ambulance to transport patient if not already in a hospital setting.

- Check pulse, blood pressure, ECG, pulse oximetry, conscious state.

- Obtain IV access

- If hypotensive, give IV normal saline 20 ml/kg rapidly and consider additional wide bore IV access.

- If required at any time, commence CPR. (cardiopulmonary resuscitation)

- Additional measures to consider if IV adrenaline infusion is ineffective.

For upper airway obstruction	• Nebulized adrenaline (5 ml e.g., 5 ampoules of 1:1000). • Consider need for advanced airway management if skills and equipment are available.
For persistent hypotension/ shock	• Give normal saline (maximum of 50ml/kg in first 30 minutes). • Glucagon
For persistent wheeze	Bronchodilators: Salbutamol 8-12 puffs of 100μg (spacer) or 5mg (nebuliser). Corticosteroids: Oral prednisolone 1 mg/kg (maximum of 50 mg) or intravenous hydrocortisone 5 mg/kg (maximum of 200 mg).

- Do not allow the patient to stand or walk until they are hemodynamically stable, which is usually a minimum of 1 hour after 1 dose of adrenaline and 4 hours if more than 1 dose of adrenaline.

- **Observe patient for at least 4 hours after last dose of adrenaline.**

- Educate the patient about anaphylaxis, risk of recurrence, trigger avoidance, self-injectable epinephrine, and thresholds for further care, and they should be referred to an allergist for follow-up evaluation.

SECTION 10
REFERENCES

REFERENCES

1. *Interventional Pain Management Image guided procedures.* Second Edition (2008). P Prithvi Raj, Lou, Erdine, Staats, Waldman, Racz, Hammer, Niv, Ruiz-Lopez and Heavner. Philadelphia, PA; Saunders Elsevier.

2. *Interventional Pain Management, A Practical Approach.* Second Edition (2016). Dwarkadas Baheti, Sanjay Bakshi, Sanjeeva Gupta and Raghbir Singh Gehdoo. New Delhi; Jaypee Brothers Medical publishers Ltd.

3. *Waldman Atlas of Interventional Pain Management.* Fourth edition (2015). Waldman SD. Philadelphia, PA; Elsevier.

4. American Society of Regional Anesthesia and Pain Medicine, https://www.asra.com/advisory-guidelines/article/3/local-anesthetic-systemic-toxicity

5. Australian Society of Clinical Immunology and Allergy Guidelines Acute management of anaphylaxis https://www.allergy.org.au/hp/papers/acute-management-of-anaphylaxis-guidelines

Get Your Surprise Gift

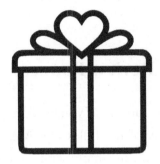

Thank you for reading this book. To show my appreciation, I've prepared a special gift for all my readers that will help you write great procedure notes. The gift is in the form of electronic templates, procedure videos, training courses, and lots more...

Access it by visiting: **https://medmantra.com/ippt**

Review Request

Reviews are like gold for authors. If you liked this book, please leave me an honest review on any of the following: Amazon, Barnes & Noble, Pothi.com, and Goodreads, or simply send me your personal feedback. I would be so happy.

Link to review URL: **https://medmantra.com/ippt**

About this book

Documentation is an integral part of clinical practice but is often neglected as it is time-consuming. This book will help you get a head start with templates that contain all the basics you need.

The book begins with a section on general considerations. Subsequent sections discuss commonly performed procedures on spine, knee, hip, abdomen & pelvis, chest & shoulder, & head, face & neck. Many techniques & approaches exist for each procedure. Sincere efforts have been taken to include all the routinely performed ones. Alternative therapies are included, which make the book comprehensive. The last section provides useful information about consent form, resuscitation, & emergency care of anaphylaxis.

This book is written to provide a practical guide *to write procedure-notes* & to serve as a *'quick revision' before* performing interventional pain procedures.

With more than 60 chapters across nine sections & an easy-to-follow presentation, this book is a useful resource for all interventional pain physicians, whether they are just embarking on training or are well established in their career.

About the author

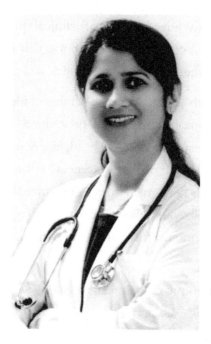

Dr. Priya Sadawarte, MBBS, MD, DNB, runs Dr. Priya's Pain Management Center at Nagpur, Maharashtra, India.

She graduated from Lokmanya Tilak Municipal Medical College & Sion Hospital, Mumbai, & then completed post-graduation in Anesthesiology from the prestigious GS Medical College & KEM Hospital, Mumbai. She has also completed DNB Anesthesiology. She then pursued advanced training in Interventional Pain Management from Mumbai & Delhi. She has published various articles in national & international peer-reviewed journals.

A dedicated teacher with teaching experience spanning over 14 years, she has been a source of eternal inspiration & motivation.

This book is her dream project to provide a practical guide to write procedure-notes precisely & effortlessly.

Made in United States
Orlando, FL
19 August 2023

36234100R00055